TELL ME THE
TRUTH,
DOCTOR

TELL ME THE
TRUTH,
DOCTOR

EASY-TO-UNDERSTAND
ANSWERS TO YOUR MOST CONFUSING
AND CRITICAL HEALTH QUESTIONS

RICHARD BESSER, M.D.

WITH JEANNE BESSER

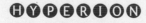

NEW YORK

Copyright © 2013 Richard Besser, M.D.

Library of Congress Cataloging-in-Publication Data

Besser, Richard.
    Tell me the truth, doctor: easy-to-understand answers to your most confusing and critical health questions/Richard Besser, MD with Jeanne Besser.—First edition.
        pages cm.
    Summary: "A book by Dr. Richard Besser of *Good Morning America*, who will give advice on how to live a longer, healthier life"—Provided by publisher.
    ISBN 978-1-4013-2483-4 (hardback)
    1. Longevity—Miscellanea.   2. Health—Miscellanea.   I. Besser, Jeanne.   II. Title.
    RA776.75.B473 2012
    613.2—dc23

                                  2012046250

Book design by Renato Stanisic

FIRST EDITION

10 9 8 7 6 5 4 3 2 1

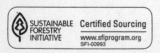

THIS LABEL APPLIES TO TEXT STOCK

We try to produce the most beautiful books possible, and we are also extremely concerned about the impact of our manufacturing process on the forests of the world and the environment as a whole. Accordingly, we've made sure that all of the paper we use has been certified as coming from forests that are managed, to ensure the protection of the people and wildlife dependent upon them.

CONTENTS

Chapter 4   Medicine Cabinet: Friend or Foe?
Your Questions on Vitamins, Supplements, and Medications 125

Chapter 5   An Ounce of Prevention, A Pound of Cure:
Your Questions for Understanding, Preventing, and Responding to Illness and Injury 167

TELL ME THE
TRUTH,
DOCTOR

INTRODUCTION

"Hey, Doc, got a minute?"

No matter where I am, a day doesn't go by without someone stopping me with that question. Sometimes the "ask" is for themselves. Other times it's for a friend or relative. Underlying all of these questions, however, is the same fundamental desire: A truthful answer from someone they trust. "Is that new diet as good as they say? Do I really need to exercise thirty minutes every day? If I have high cholesterol, should I go on a statin? How do I find the best doctor?" These questions may sound straightforward, but with all the conflicting information you hear about every day, it's hard to know what to do.

Being able to deliver medical information with a personal touch means a lot to me. I come from a long line of doctors whose patients were like family. House calls weren't unheard-of and offering assistance took precedence over everything else. I think most of us are nostalgic for the days when we thought nothing of picking up the phone to talk to our physician if we had a concern. Now it can take days to get a return phone call, and it's rarely from the doctor you wanted to reach. Feeling discouraged and disconnected, you may try to self-diagnose and end up spending even more money on expensive supplements or treatments that don't work. Instead of throwing that money away, let me give you—in this book—that house call you've been missing so that you can truly make informed decisions about your health.

I will provide easy-to-understand answers to many of your most critical and confusing health questions. My goal is to help you discover what you need to do to feel better now and to live a longer, healthier life. Throughout the book, I will provide tools to teach you how to separate the truth from the clutter and will explain why perception is so often different from reality. I guess I find it easy to tell the truth because I view health quite simply. There's no secret formula to staying well. Health isn't something given to you by a doctor. It doesn't come in a medicine bottle. Health comes to you incrementally over time, and it leaves you in the same way. It happens through a series of choices you make dozens of times each day, choices about what you do and what you ignore. It can be something as small as deciding between a side salad or fries. Taking the stairs instead of the elevator. Hitting the gym instead of hitting the snooze button. It can be more challenging, like telling your doctor you don't want to take a test he's recommending. Asking for a second opinion instead of automatically accepting a diagnosis. Saying no to taking a supplement your friend swears by. All of these actions, big and small, have an impact on your well-being.

You are constantly barraged by experts offering another approach to health, usually the quick fix. It comes in many guises: A new pill to swallow, a new diet or supplement to try. That isn't how you achieve health, and it isn't how you maintain it. But being healthy doesn't have to be hard, either. It just takes understanding the choices you are already making and deciding if you really want to make a change. I want to empower you to own your health, to seek the truth, and to trust your instincts.

I know how hard it can be to navigate the health care system. I too have had the challenges of finding a new doctor, overcoming a disabling medical condition, and watching a loved one die from a medical error. As a parent, I worry about my teenage sons and whether they will make the right decisions for their own well-being. As a pediatrician, I focus on helping my patients understand the underpinnings of health, so they can make informed choices for themselves and their children. And as the Chief

Medical Editor at ABC News, I have the responsibility to clearly state my opinion on the critical health challenges of our time to millions of Americans. Every day, new studies pass my desk with banner headlines of medical breakthroughs. Cures for this disease. Ways to stop another. I wish they were all true, but from experience I know to be skeptical. One day eggs are good for you, the next day they aren't, and then they are again. Why? Unfortunately, sometimes medicine is predicated on partial truths, or as Stephen Colbert calls it, "truthiness." If being vitamin deficient is bad for your health (and clearly it is), shouldn't taking extra vitamins be good for you? A whole vitamin and supplement industry is built on that bit of "truthiness," and Congress is responsible for letting them do it unabatedly. That doesn't mean it's the right thing for you.

How do you know what to believe? It's not easy. The reality is that today more than ever, medicine is a business as well as a calling. It is critical to understand when the health care industry crosses the line, as more services are being pushed for profit rather than your benefit. How does this affect your perception of the truth? Just turn on the television. There are constant advertisements from pharmaceutical, weight loss, and supplement industries barraging you with images of happy, healthy, smiling people enjoying their products. It's government assaulted by special interest groups' and lobbyists' dollars, hoping to sway policies. How can government regulatory agencies solely focus on the health of the public with these corrupting influences? It's the power of HMOs to pressure medical personnel to be more efficient, even if that means taking less time with their patients—a lot less time. And then there are medical research and science. How do you interpret the latest information when some studies are designed to promote products rather than to find more objective truths? It's hard to make good health care decisions when the person giving you advice stands to make money off what you decide to do.

Corporate, government, and institutional malfeasance aren't the only barriers to overcome. Even your most well-meaning friends, neighbors, and colleagues can be stumbling blocks on the road to better health. Every winter I hear the same complaint from people at work: "I got the flu shot once and it gave me the flu. I'm never getting that shot again." Before I know it, half of my office is eschewing the vaccine. As hard as I try, no amount of data can budge that firmly held opinion. How a vaccine that doesn't contain any live virus can cause the flu is beyond me, but for some things, "the truth" is based on personal experience. More and more frequently, these anecdotal beliefs are trumping science. It is harder and harder for the untrained eye to sort out the good from the bad.

Why do I care so much? It's because there were so many inspirational people who believed in me and set an example for me to follow. My grandfather was a family doctor and my grandmother was his nurse well into their eighties. They were my idols. My grandfather would always give me logic problems to work out and taught me that medicine combined the mental challenge of figuring things out with the joy of helping people. My grandmother, an immigrant via Ellis Island, taught me the importance of hard work and instilled in me a strong sense of right and wrong—a moral thread that forms the backbone of my approach to medicine and to life.

I was the third generation in my family to go to medical school at the University of Pennsylvania. When I went to the children's hospital for my first rotation in pediatrics, I knew that I had found my calling. Here was a field of medicine that spoke to my heart. It focused on prevention: How do you help parents raise children who will live long and healthy lives? The concepts seemed so straightforward. Prevent disease and promote health. Simple in concept, but not always as easy to put into practice.

When I was a pediatric resident at Johns Hopkins Hospital, my chairman was Frank Oski. A brilliant man, he inspired me to pursue medicine as a field of inquiry. He wanted me, and everyone he trained, not just to practice medicine, but to move the field forward. Ask questions and when you found one without a good answer, do the research to get that answer. He taught me not to accept a way of practicing medicine without understanding why. He never seemed quite as happy as when he was debunking a myth or challenging the status quo. The year I spent as his chief resident infected me with that same passion.

After training in pediatrics, I chose a career in public health while continuing to practice pediatrics part-time. For me it was an easy career choice. As a doctor I got to interact with and have an impact on the health of my patients, one at a time, but as a public health practitioner, I got to do much more. In public health all the people of the world are our patients. By understanding what causes disease and by developing and implementing prevention programs as a public health doctor, I got to improve the lives of entire populations.

In 2009, when I was acting director of the Centers for Disease Control and Prevention, an influenza pandemic broke out. As part of the response, I took to the airways every morning and evening for the news broadcasts. I also held a press conference every afternoon to talk about the state of the outbreak and the response. People were scared, and rightfully so. The communication principle I applied, taught to me at CDC, was simple: Tell the truth. Tell people what you know as soon as you know it. If you don't know the answer, say so, and then say what you are going to do to get the answers. So simple, but so rarely done. It was my experience during the pandemic response—engendering trust by telling the truth in straightforward language—that led me to take the job as Chief Medical Editor at ABC News. My idea was to see if I could practice public health through the power and reach of our network.

So now, every day at ABC News, as I prepare to do a report, I sift through the medical literature to find "the story behind the story." I look at the research to see what the science says. Usually there are conflicting studies. If I am going to recommend something or give my opinion, I want to know the evidence. I then want to know how the experts in a particular field interpret the same information. Do they agree or disagree? Do they feel there is enough evidence to recommend that people change their behaviors based on the current information? And when I hear experts give opinions, I want to know what they are based on and whether they have any conflict of interest. Are they receiving money from someone who could benefit from the outcome of the study? This information doesn't make me discount their opinions, but it allows me to interpret them through the right filter. This is how I was trained. Always ask questions and always question dogma. In the end, translate all this information into common-sense, straightforward advice that you can use.

The inquisitorial skills that I use for every story are the same ones I use to answer the questions you will find on these pages. Many topics reflect on the everyday concerns about diet and exercise, two of the fundamentals of good health. I'll explore what works, what doesn't, and why. I'll also combat the common myths and misperceptions that pervade our lives, everything from how to fall asleep to whether you can catch a cold from going out in the cold with wet hair. I'll also take a good look at your medicine cabinet and tell you what you need, when you need it, and what to do with everything else. The more you know and understand about your health, the more it will empower you to make difficult decisions that are best for you. Understanding the nature of diseases and your risks of contracting them will allow you to be more involved in your health care choices and improve your relationship with your doctor, a relationship that is at the core of your well-being.

Throughout the book I'll be talking a lot about risk and risk factors. These are terms that are used so much when it comes to health. I'll talk about different kinds of risk. There are certain risk factors that you can't do anything about, for instance those you inherit. I'll explain why it's important to know about these even though you can't change them. Knowing you are at increased risk for certain diseases may help motivate you to focus on changing certain behaviors to minimize those risks, and it will definitely help your doctor guide your health decisions. Most of the focus, though, will be on what are called modifiable risk factors, those things you can do something about. I'll be blunt about the consequences of risky health behavior, but I'll also make the changes as easy to handle as possible. Once you are successful at making the first small change to improve your health, you'll be hooked. It only gets easier and easier.

This book will give you the information you need to start improving your health today, but pace yourself. There's too much information to take in at once. My wife is a cookbook writer. No one reads a cookbook from cover to cover at once. I think that the approach to this book should be the same. A little at a time. Let your glance drift to something that catches your eye and read a question or two. Put it down and the next time you pick it up, another issue might be of more interest. Every answer ends with an easy-to-digest summary called Dr. B's Bottom Line. Sprinkled throughout are sidebars that give you more quick tips for improving your health. Many topics offer changes you can implement right away to improve your health. Pick an easy one. Then put the book down for a week or two. Make that change and focus on sticking to it. If you were one of my pediatric patients I would say keep a calendar and give yourself a star every day you do it. After a bit of time, if you are still doing it, give yourself a big pat on the back and move on to the next change. It's the key to success. Start small and savor the incredible feeling you'll get as you head down the road to better health. And don't forget to look in the back for references, resources, and information that will help you along your way.

1

DROP THAT FRENCH FRY AND NO ONE GETS HURT

Your Questions on Diets, Nutrition, and Food Safety

I get more questions about diets than just about any other subject. It's easy to see why. We are a nation obsessed with eating as well as with losing weight. We are bombarded with food ads showing happy, attractive, thin people chowing down on mega-meals. The result: We're one of the fattest nations on earth.

You know that being overweight isn't good for your health. Most of us want to take the extra pounds off, and we want to do it as fast and as painlessly as possible. There's an entire weight loss industry happy to supply you with a variety of products and methods claiming to help you do just that. Most of these are fad diets that deprive you of calories in a big way, at least early on. In doing so, the pounds may come off quickly. However, these diets aren't sustainable, so the pounds slowly return. Overeating followed by over-restricting becomes an endless cycle that profits those who make money by selling diet foods and weight loss plans. But it is a terrible approach to health.

It's easy to see why failure is common. Many of us have a complicated relationship with food. From the time we were young, food wasn't just sustenance. It was comfort. It was a reward. It was a way of showing love. Withholding food was a form of punishment. When we were bad, it was "No dessert for you." If we didn't finish our meals, we were told, "There are children starving in China," and we remained at the table until the plate was clean. It's no wonder we're so conflicted about enjoying food without overeating and feel guilty for stopping when we are full.

Learning how to unload this baggage will allow you to make better decisions about which foods to choose. Foods shouldn't be categorized as "good" or "bad." There are clearly some foods that work best as "every-day" foods and some foods that are better as "sometimes" foods, but we tend to get into trouble when certain foods are labeled "never" foods. The temptation can just be too great. How do you get that balance between these types of food? This is a theme you will see running through many of the questions and answers in this chapter.

Dietary changes should not just be about losing weight, though. Choosing foods higher in fiber and lower in fat, salt, and sugar helps prevent heart disease, diabetes, and cancer. And the benefits of better eating choices can help the next generation, too. One of the most common concerns from my patients' parents is how to get their kids to kick their junk food habit. I tell them it starts with them. Setting a good example is paramount to their children's success.

The truth is this: You have to decide that you *want* to live a longer, more robust life. Maintaining a healthy weight is the first step. But it can't be done with a quick fix. The only route to success is making long-term diet and lifestyle changes. I'm not asking you to give up anything. Healthy eating is about making simple choices and simple changes that you can live with. Follow the principles in this section and you'll see how to do it. Remember, start small, experience success, and build from there. The little sustainable changes you make add up over time to major weight loss and improved health.

1

ARE DIETS THE BEST WAY TO LOSE WEIGHT?

A couple of years ago I did a segment for *Good Morning America* in which I presented a panel of nutritionists with some of the latest, hottest celebrity diets: A raw food diet, a blood-type diet, a macrobiotic diet, and the master cleanse. Their job was to tell me which was the best, which was the worst, and which might be downright dangerous. I knew what *I* thought were the correct answers, but I wanted to see if they agreed. Turns out they did.

All of the diets resulted in weight loss for a simple reason: They restricted calories. Some eliminated whole categories of food; others used pseudoscience to tell you what to eat. While a macrobiotic diet can be a healthy approach to eating if done carefully, none of the diets was a healthy approach to weight loss. I view a diet as a "quick fix" when you need to lose an extra pound or two after a weekend splurge or to kick-start swimsuit season. As a long-term approach to weight loss diets just don't work. You can't stick to them forever, and with some diets it would be dangerous to do so.

The diet industry is huge, and Americans spend billions of dollars a year trying to lose weight. For some reason we continue to believe that the answer to losing extra pounds has got to be the newest diet book or product. When that fails, we try the next one. The result is yo-yo dieting or weight cycling: Your weight goes down due to severe, unsustainable caloric restrictions and then it comes back up, usually to a point higher than where you started.

This country is in the middle of a health crisis. More than one-third of adults are obese. Another third of adults are overweight but not yet obese. The impact on our health is deadly: Heart disease, stroke, type 2 diabetes, and certain types of cancer, all increased by obesity.

I firmly believe that the only meaningful way to lose weight is to make long-term changes to your eating habits and incorporate more activity into your days. It all starts with small steps. Even a modest weight loss will provide important health benefits. Don't get discouraged if it takes a while to see dramatic results. Chances are you have put on your extra weight over the course of years. It could take that long to get it all off.

There are a million weight loss strategies; you can check them all out on the Internet. For me it boils down to three rules:

- Eat less.
- Eat differently.
- Move more.

There's nothing fancy or complicated. This isn't a short-term change where you eat something crazy for a week. It isn't about eliminating foods you love or training to be a triathlete. It is about small, livable changes that become habits. It is as much a mental adjustment as a physical one.

Eat Less

You need food to fuel your body. Food gives you the energy to do what you need to get done. But there's no way around it—you may be eating too much. Portion size has exploded. Everything is supersized. Remember what a bagel, a muffin, or even a fast-food hamburger looked like twenty years ago? Now they are two or even three times as large. We need to get back to healthy portions and the right balance of foods.

Cut back gradually. When you serve yourself, start by taking only three-quarters of what you would normally eat. After a month or so, do that again. Fill your plate with veggies and whole grains first, then add lean protein. Learn to eat only when you're hungry. How many times have you gorged yourself only to think, "I didn't even really need that"? Be conscious of when you are eating and learn your triggers for overeating—for some it's boredom, for others stress.

Don't be afraid to use a visual reminder. Put a big sign on your refrigerator—"Stop. Are you really hungry?" or tack up a photo of yourself at a former weight or someone at a weight you want to achieve for inspiration. Maybe you have a goal. Put a picture of someone doing an activity you hope to do, an athlete you admire, or a reward, like an outfit you want to fit into. Motivation comes in all forms.

Eating is also a social activity and no one wants to give up those get-togethers. Unfortunately, research shows that most of us eat more when we're with others than when we are by ourselves. Find additional ways to socialize, preferably ones built around physical activity. Even going to a movie or strolling around the mall with a friend is better than always meeting for drinks and nachos.

The number of calories *you* need depends on your size and your amount of activity. Two helpful tools for assessing your needs are the Centers for Disease Control and Prevention's adult BMI calculator, www.cdc.gov /healthyweight/assessing/bmi, and the U.S. Department of Agriculture's ChooseMyPlate.gov site, which offers the new governmental food guidelines to help you make healthier choices, www.choosemyplate.gov/weight -management-calories.html.

Keep a diet diary and then go online to figure out how many calories you are consuming right now. Then look at ways to make a change. If you take in five hundred calories less each day than you burn up, you will lose around a pound per week, a realistic goal. This can be split between eating a bit less and exercising a bit more.

Eat Differently

In a 2007 *New York Times* article, the food writer Michael Pollan gave simple but accurate advice: "Eat food. Not too much. Mostly plants." I couldn't agree with him more. Eat food your great-grandmother would recognize— fruits, vegetables, and products with ingredients you don't need a degree in chemistry to understand. Start fresh. I like to say there are no bad foods, but I make one exception: Soda. Get rid of it. Sure, you can have one occasionally, but best to get it out of the house so it's not there to tempt you. It's just empty calories that have absolutely no nutritional value. Cut back on other sweetened beverages. Say good-bye to the chips and all the other junk food that is going to sideline you. I'm not saying you should never eat processed food, but if you don't keep it around, it will be easier to regulate. Save it for a treat when you are dining out. You'll also be less tempted to indulge if it's not in your cupboard. You might need to "retrain" your palate to enjoy less sugary and salty snacks. Replace junk food with healthier options. Instead of processed food snacks, keep dried fruit and nuts for munching. Keep a bag of baby carrots in the fridge but get rid of the ranch dressing.

These steps aren't easy to do, so here's my advice: Do it gradually. As a pediatrician, I often help parents wean their toddlers off juices. We start by mixing the juice with a little bit of water, then gradually increase the water and lessen the juice. After a month or so, the children are drinking water and enjoying it. You can go the same route. Gradually wean yourself from sodas, juices, and snack foods. If it's too hard for you to eat a sandwich without chips, try the baked variety and eat half of what you normally would. I like to put a serving on my plate and put away the bag so I'm not tempted to go back for more. Fill up your plate with a side salad, carrots, or sliced apples, so you don't feel deprived. Trade half-and-half in your coffee for milk, and go from full-fat dairy to lower-fat options.

Move More

I'm not even going to say exercise more. Just move. Take the stairs. Go for a walk—two or three times a day if you can, even for five to ten minutes: Before you start your day, at lunch, and after work. It doesn't have to be far, but just start somewhere. Once you are walking for a while, try seeing if you can walk faster, longer, or even jog a little. Ask a friend to go with you. Join a gym. Get a trainer, anything to get you to stick to it. That's all it takes, little steps that become bigger ones.

Changing your lifestyle to lose weight permanently is not going to be easy. You are not going to be perfect. You shouldn't be. Just forgive yourself and get back on track if you get derailed. Food is something we should enjoy. Losing weight will never work if you equate it with punishment. Think of all the benefits of being healthier, instead of fixating on what you are giving up. It's all about balance.

DR. B'S BOTTOM LINE:

Dieting is not the best way to lose weight. Unfortunately, there is no magic to weight loss. To lose pounds and to keep them off, you need to make a lifetime commitment to get your weight under control through healthy choices. Eat less, eat healthier foods, and move more. Your body will thank you for it.

MY TOP 3 TIPS FOR LOSING WEIGHT

CAN THE SODAS

Replace your daily twenty-ounce soda with water and you could lose twenty-five pounds in a year, or try sparkling water with a splash of juice instead.

TAKE IT HOME

It is so hard to watch what you eat when you dine out. Restaurant portions have ballooned. At the start of the meal, ask for a takeout container and only leave on your plate what you want to eat. It is harder to resist overeating if you wait until the end of the meal to pack it to go.

BUY NEW PLACE SETTINGS

Studies show that people take smaller portions if they are given smaller plates and bowls. Look in your cupboard and think about downsizing. Also, color matters. If you serve your food on plates that contrast with the food color, your portion will look larger and you will eat less.

2

WILL EATING SIX SMALL MEALS A DAY INSTEAD OF THREE BIG ONES HELP ME LOSE WEIGHT?

Six meals instead of three? As my kids would say, "Sweet!" Who wouldn't want to eat twice as often? Why stop at six? Eight is even better. Or is it?

With all the diet books and various weight loss strategies, it is so hard to convince my patients that losing weight is all about taking in fewer calories than you burn off. It doesn't matter if you eat three meals or ten—if you consume the same total number of calories and types of food over the course of the day, your weight loss or gain will be the same.

What got everyone talking was a 2001 study in the *British Medical Journal* that found that people who reported eating six small meals each day had lower cholesterol than those who said they ate one or two. Suddenly experts were weighing in on why smaller meals were better. Some supposed they helped to keep your metabolism revved up. Others thought with constant grazing, overeating from hunger would be less likely than when you had a longer span between meals. But when all was said and done, there was no consensus on whether you were metabolically better off eating three or six meals.

A 2010 study finally addressed this head-on. Two groups went on a weight loss plan, consuming the same calories. One group ate three meals and the other ate six. At the end of the study, there was no statistical difference between the amounts of weight lost by the two groups.

Now, I do need to throw a bit of a wrench in the works when it comes to "a calorie is just a calorie." There are new data that suggest the type of calorie does have some impact on how you burn it, by changing something called your metabolic rate. The higher your metabolic rate, both while exercising and at rest, the more calories you will burn up. Ever know someone who can eat as much as he wants and never gain weight? This may be due to his metabolic rate being higher. Researchers at Harvard studied people on three types of diets of equal calories: A low-fat diet, a low-carbohydrate diet, and a diet low in fat but rich in complex carbohydrates. They found that those on the traditional American Heart Association low-fat diet had the biggest drop in their metabolic rate. They just did not burn up calories as fast. Those on the low-carb diet had the smallest drop, with those on the complex carbohydrates in between. While they didn't follow people long term, this suggests that what type of food you eat—in addition to the total number of calories—may have an impact on how easy it is to lose weight and keep it off. Stay tuned, as this is a hot area for ongoing research.

But back to six meals. I'm not saying that this style of eating is wrong or harmful. The important thing is finding what works for you. If you frequently get hungry, or are afraid of being deprived while losing weight, having smaller "meals" might work better for you. Remember, these six "meals" should each have about half the calories of traditional meals. They should also be nutritionally balanced. For others, such a small meal is just not satisfying.

DR. B'S BOTTOM LINE:

Assuming you eat the same types of food and take in the same number of calories over the course of the day, whether you eat six small meals a day or three larger traditional meals, you will gain or lose the same amount of weight.

SNACK TIME

Here are my favorite healthy, well-balanced mini-meals. Try one the next time you're hungry.
- Cheese, apple slices, and whole wheat crackers
- Peanut butter on a banana with raisins

- Hummus on whole-wheat pita and carrot sticks
- Greek yogurt, fruit, and granola parfait
- Half a whole-wheat bagel with tuna salad and tomato
- Half a turkey, avocado, and tomato sandwich on multigrain bread
- Multigrain waffle with almond butter and strawberry slices
- Smoothie made with yogurt, frozen fruit, and fruit juice
- Quesadilla with cheese, black beans, chopped veggies, and salsa

3

ARE JUICE FASTS GOOD FOR ME?

My wife is a yoga enthusiast. At her favorite yoga studio, not a month goes by without someone sponsoring a juice fast. When she's asked if she'll participate, she replies, "No thanks." She, like I, believes that eating sensibly is the best way to stay healthy and maintain a desired weight. When she questions her fellow yoginis why they are partaking or asks what they know about the actual product, she's usually met by silence or phrases like "flushing toxins" and "cleansing systems." No one really knows why they are shelling out hundreds of dollars *not* to eat, instead of spending a fraction of that amount buying healthful foods.

Fad diets, including cleanses, seem to be contagious. You hear of celebrities dropping scores of pounds for a role by drinking some horrifying lemon and cayenne pepper concoction and think, "Well I can do that, if I will look like them." I'm not sure why many dieters are willing to go to those extremes, but when it comes to maintaining healthful eating habits, day in and day out, it seems too difficult.

The Academy of Nutrition and Dietetics (formerly the American Dietetic Association) recommends staying away from fad diets. If you lose weight too quickly, you'll lose muscle, bone, and water and be more likely to regain the pounds quickly afterward.

The argument for juice fasts relies on two important misconceptions: That our digestive system needs a reprieve from solid foods and that nutrients in liquids can be more easily absorbed than solids. There is no scientific data to back either rationale. Unless you have a problem with your digestive system that prevents you from breaking down solid food, there is no need for a liquid diet.

When it comes to toxins, your body has quite wonderful systems for handling them. Your kidneys and liver work to remove and excrete them through bodily waste. Some toxins get deposited in your bones and other tissues and take time to be excreted. However, there is nothing to suggest that drinking liquids helps liberate these toxins from your body any faster. Similarly, colonics do not cleanse your colon any better than normal digestive function and in fact, can cause injury if incorrectly done.

A juice fast isn't even guaranteed to make you lose weight. If the juices are low-calorie, you will lose weight, but some juices have added sweeteners, which could actually deliver the opposite effect. You will lose or gain the same amount of weight, calorie for calorie, whether you ingest it as a liquid or as a solid. By juicing your fruits and vegetables you are also losing out on the nutrients found in the skin and pulp and are more likely to feel hungry *faster* because you are missing the fiber. There's just no good reason not to simply eat what you think you are drinking. That way you know exactly what you are ingesting and you're doing it in its purest, unadulterated form. Another reason to look at the ingredients: Some cleanses contain supplements and herbal products that can be dangerous.

As always, the best medical advice for losing weight is to eat a diet based on vegetables, fruits, whole grains, and lean sources of protein. Choose water to stay hydrated.

DR. B'S BOTTOM LINE:

Juice fasts are not good for you. Effective weight loss is done through moderation, not through extreme diets focusing on short-term gains. Let your body do what it's designed to do. It really functions quite well! You don't need gimmicks like liquid diets to lose weight, and there is nothing to suggest that your organs need a rest. If you feel like eating lighter, concentrate on eating more fruits and vegetables. The fiber will fill you up and keep you from overeating.

4

CAN EATING TOO MUCH SUGAR CAUSE DIABETES?

When I was at the CDC and even now at ABC News, I've often been asked what health issues keep me up at night. I would say the one medical condition that really concerns me is diabetes. In the United States today, almost twenty-six million people live with diabetes, a chronic disease that can impact almost every organ in your body. It can cause kidney failure, vascular disease, nerve damage, heart disease, and blindness. According to the American Diabetes Association, diabetes was responsible for more than seventy-one thousand deaths in 2007. The CDC predicts that as many as one in three American adults will have diabetes by 2050 unless there is a concerted effort to curb obesity and get more active.

For many, the first thing that comes to mind at the mention of diabetes is high blood sugar. The notion that eating too much sugar directly contributes to diabetes seems logical for a number of reasons. Those living with diabetes must eat sweet treats sparingly and consistently monitor their blood sugar levels in order to keep them within a safe range.

So is eating too much sugar going to lead to diabetes? First let's look a bit at the disease; there are actually several different types of diabetes, each having different causes and risk factors:

- **Type 1 diabetes** is also known as juvenile-onset diabetes because it primarily strikes children and young adults. It develops when your body's immune system destroys the cells located in your pancreas that make insulin. It isn't clear why this happens; it may be triggered by certain infections and it may also be inherited. Insulin is a hormone with many functions but for the purposes of this discussion it regulates how your body uses glucose. Without insulin, your body's cells cannot use the sugar in your bloodstream for energy and it builds up. As a result, type 1 diabetics must take insulin injections.

- **Type 2 diabetes** is also known as non-insulin-dependent diabetes mellitus. With this disease, your pancreas still makes insulin but there is a problem in how your cells use it. They become resistant to its effects, leading to a buildup of sugar in your blood. We used to call it adult-onset diabetes because it primarily affected adults but we don't use that term anymore as it is now being seen more and more often in children. There is a strong connection between type 2 diabetes and obesity and physical inactivity. Both are big risk factors. Left untreated it usually progresses with symptoms beginning gradually, sometimes imperceptibly for years. The good news: If you catch it early, changes in diet and exercise may be able to control it. Ninety-five percent of people with diabetes have type 2.
- **Gestational diabetes** is diabetes that occurs during pregnancy. Like type 2, there is a link with obesity, ethnicity, and family history. For most women, their blood sugar returns to normal soon after delivery but some develop diabetes five to ten years after childbirth, so it is important to continue to be closely monitored. Its treatment is similar to that for type 2 diabetes.

Type 1 diabetes has no link with diet and weight. With type 2 diabetes, obesity, combined with physical inactivity and genetics, is the chief determinant. But the direct relationship of sugar as a major contributor to diabetes remains largely unsupported. The American Diabetes Association puts this in the category of myth, and I think that is right. The ADA believes that it doesn't matter whether those extra calories come from excess sugar, fat, or just overeating. It's all the calories put together that play a role.

Some researchers aren't so sure. A number of studies have shown an association between the amount of sugary drinks people consume and their risk of developing diabetes. However, most people who overdo it on sugar are also overdoing it on calories.

DR. B'S BOTTOM LINE:

If you are worried about developing diabetes, worry less about eating too much sugar and concentrate more on achieving a healthy weight by eating a balanced diet and getting regular exercise.

SNEAKY AND SWEET

Use caution if equating sugar-free or sweetened with agar or honey as being lower-caloric or more healthful options when choosing treats—they often aren't. Make sure to read labels to see what you are getting.

5

SHOULD I DRINK EIGHT GLASSES OF WATER A DAY?

Anyone who's been on a diet has heard the advice, "Drink eight glasses of water a day." The theory was partially based on water filling you up to prevent you from overeating. You could always tell who was following that dictate—they were never far from the bathroom. The "8 × 8" maxim (eight, eight-ounce glasses) has been espoused as the solution not just for losing weight, but for everything from supermodel-worthy glowing skin to regulating the digestive system by "flushing out toxins."

Before we go any further, let me say, I love water. Drinking water is a great thing. I wish all my patients named water, instead of soda, fruit juice, or sports drinks, as their beverage of choice. But even with my ringing endorsement, water, like everything, is best in moderation. This isn't denying the important role that water plays in keeping our bodies functioning properly. You can live without food for far longer than you can without water. But with a normal diet, the truth is, your body does a really good job of regulating your need for liquids, primarily by letting you know when you're thirsty!

Here's why. One of the main functions of your kidneys is to preserve the water and salt balance in your blood. They keep the concentration of salts within a very narrow range. When you drink extra water that might dilute out these salts, your kidneys get rid of the excess water into your urine. At these times you may notice your urine is paler. When you are not drinking as much, your kidneys react by holding on to more water. Your urine gets concentrated and appears darker (and a little more pungent). Whether you are drinking eight glasses of water a day or twenty glasses, your kidneys will do their job.

The magic number eight can be traced back to 1945, when the U.S. Food and Nutrition Board, part of the Institutes of Medicine, provided guidelines for good nutrition. They calculated this figure based on the amount of water needed to break down and use your food. In the most recently published guidelines in 2004, the U.S. National Research Council increased the recommendation slightly to 2.7 liters of water for women and 3.7 liters for men. Translating liters to eight-ounce glasses, this comes out to eleven glasses for women and fifteen glasses for men. Nearly a gallon for men! How's that possible? The guidelines note a couple of important details: Healthy people adequately meet their daily hydration needs by letting thirst be their guide. This means if you have a normal thirst mechanism and access to water, you don't need to think about how much water you need to drink. You will drink enough. Another key point is that the water recommendations include all the water you consume. For an average diet, food provides 20 percent of your daily water needs. If you eat a lot of fruits and vegetables, you are getting even more water. Most fruits and vegetables are more than 80 percent water. Even meats have water. Cooked chicken, for example, is actually 60 percent water.

How much water you should drink really depends on your level of activity, how hot and humid it is outside, and what you eat throughout the day. As your activity level increases or you lose water through sweating and evaporation, thirst kicks in, and tells you to drink. Most of us anticipate these losses by drinking extra when we know we may have a chance of getting dehydrated.

As a doctor, there are many times I recommend that patients increase their fluid intake when they are sick. When I see someone with a cold I know that if they have a little fever and rapid breathing, they will lose extra water. However, I have to tell you, there are no studies that show increasing fluid intake will make you get better sooner. This is one of those recommendations based on experience and scientific principles rather than studies. In fact a review in the *British Medical Journal* suggests that increasing fluids when you have a respiratory infection may be harmful. I disagree with their conclusion, but it points out how something you have taken as the gospel may not have a lot of evidence behind it.

I do think drinking water rather than other beverages makes a lot of sense. There isn't a lot of data to show that water itself helps you lose weight, but if you are substituting water for high-calorie drinks, it sure helps. It is the first thing I recommend to any patient who wants to cut back on calories.

DR. B'S BOTTOM LINE:

Your body actually needs more than eight glasses of water a day, but you don't really need to think about it. Your brain and kidneys take care of that for you. Trust your body to signal when you need to drink more. That is what thirst is all about. Rather than counting glasses, look at what's in them. If you are drinking a lot of things other than water, think about making a change. It's one of the simplest things you can do for your health.

STRANGE BUT TRUE?

You can actually drink too much water, a situation known as water intoxication. It is mainly seen in people with altered thirst, mental illness, or where water is being provided by a feeding tube or intravenous drip. While rare, an excess amount of water can dilute the amount of sodium and other essential salts in your blood and can be fatal.

6

WILL SKIPPING BREAKFAST HELP ME LOSE WEIGHT?

In my family, I'm teased for being predictable. I prefer to say I like a routine, especially when it comes to my mornings. I begin each day the same way, with the newspaper and my coffee, orange juice, and a bowl of cereal topped with fruit—bananas and raisins in the fall and winter, berries in the spring and summer. I need to eat breakfast before I can do anything else, and as it turns out that's good for my health, too.

Many studies from around the world have shown that people who skip breakfast are more likely to be overweight. At first that might sound absurd. How can skipping a meal lead to weight gain? If weight is all about calories in and calories burned, skipping breakfast would have to decrease weight gain. However, studies show that when people skip breakfast, they are more likely to be hungry during the rest of the day and end up eating more for their other meals. Instead of saving the calories from breakfast they actually consume more total calories over the course of the day.

I find eating breakfast serves another purpose. It really improves my disposition. If I skip breakfast (or any meal, for that matter) my mood suffers. I am grumpy, can't concentrate as well, and lose my focus. I'm not alone. This has been seen in both children and adults.

So whether you are trying to watch your weight or just get your day off to the right start, begin with breakfast. For me it also serves another purpose. It gives me a little time to wake up, catch up with what is going on in the world, and take a deep breath. All of these plus I'm doing my body a favor and keeping my weight in check to boot!

DR. B'S BOTTOM LINE:

Breakfast is often called the most important meal because it gives you energy at the start of the day and helps prevent overeating during later meals. I know

it's tempting to skip it because you'd rather sleep a little longer or aren't hungry first thing in the morning. Even if you don't sit down for long, grab something to get your day off to a healthful start before leaving the house or to eat on the road.

THE FIVE-MINUTE BREAKFAST

Here's my recipe for a good breakfast: Fruit, lean protein, and complex carbohydrates, preferably ones high in fiber. Whole grains take longer for your body to digest and leave you feeling full for longer. Top the cereal with fruit and have a glass of orange juice to give you a jump start toward meeting your "five-a-day" goal.

Here are four of my favorites:

- One cup of low-fat yogurt, 1/2 cup homemade low-fat granola, fruit in season or raisins; 6 ounces of calcium-fortified orange juice; coffee with low-fat milk.
- Whole grain cereal topped with fruit in season; 1/2 grapefruit; 6 ounces of calcium-fortified orange juice; coffee with low-fat milk.
- Two fried eggs on toasted English muffin; 1/2 grapefruit; 6 ounces of calcium-fortified orange juice; coffee with low-fat milk.
- Whole-grain toast with natural peanut butter; 1/2 grapefruit; 6 ounces of calcium-fortified orange juice; coffee with low-fat milk.

7

IS BOTTLED WATER BETTER THAN TAP?

I love water. I drink it all the time: Plain water, bubbly water. It doesn't matter. I even ask all of my patients about water: "Do you drink it? How much?"

My friend Rosemary also loves water. Whenever she comes to visit from out of state, her first stop on the way from the airport is to the gourmet supermarket to load up on her favorite bottled water. She's half-convinced that drinking this brand, sourced from a pristine island eight thousand miles away, will cure almost anything that ails her.

Her views are not unusual. Somehow the simplicity of water has been corrupted. Pouring some from your kitchen sink just doesn't seem good enough anymore. There's pressure to order artisan water, and the fancier the bottle the better.

The growth of bottled water in the United States over the past decade has been absolutely meteoric. In 2009, we spent more than $10 billion drinking more than eight billion gallons of the stuff. But is it really worth it? The reality is you're doing yourself *and* the environment a disservice if you're forking out big bucks for bottled water, *especially* if you are doing it because you think it's better for you. It's not—or at least there is no way to know that it is.

Here's the truth. Both tap water and bottled water are regulated, but the system for tap water has transparency and the one for bottled water does not. The Environmental Protection Agency is responsible for overseeing the quality of tap water through the Safe Drinking Water Act. They have given this authority to test and ensure community water standards to the states and territories. Every community water system with more than one hundred thousand customers is required to post their water quality information online. You can check on yours by reading a Consumer Confidence report at water.epa.gov. Bottled water is regulated by the Food and Drug Administration (FDA). However, there are no requirements that water bottlers share the results of their testing with the FDA or even use independent labs. While the FDA is required to inspect bottling facilities, they are considered low-risk producers and inspections are a rare event.

But doesn't bottled water spring from a better source, as the advertisements imply? Not necessarily. Just as in Oz, where the man behind the curtain wasn't who you thought he was, you'd be surprised to find out where most bottled water comes from. According to their websites, both Pepsi's Aquafina brand and Coca-Cola's Dasani water come from public water sources. That's right, it's just purified tap water. But tap water by law already is purified. As your grandmother might say, "Why pay for milk when you can get the cow for free?"

There is one good thing about the bottled water boom. It's gotten people into drinking water and has moved many away from sweetened drinks. For years, the lukewarm office water fountain was ignored in favor of canned sodas. Now water is cool to consume. But we have to drink it in a more environmentally responsible way. A study by the Environmental Working Group found that every twenty-seven hours Americans consume enough bottled water to circle the equator with plastic bottles stacked end to end. Worse, most of those bottles are not recycled.

Make the better decision: If you are on the go, use reusable stainless steel or BPA-free bottles. Hopefully, carrying your own water will become the status symbol of the future. If you are sensitive to the taste of your tap water or are concerned about contaminants in your local water supply, use a filter and change the cartridge regularly.

DR. B'S BOTTOM LINE:

Bottled water is not better than tap water. As you can tell, I'm quite passionate about water being your beverage of choice. So let's not make it more complicated than we need to. Save your money and the environment. Even in fast-food restaurants I ask for a cup of tap water—they are happy enough to oblige.

AND IF YOU NEED ANOTHER REASON . . .

In addition to more transparent testing, most bottled water doesn't offer what the CDC named as one of the ten great public health achievements of the twentieth century: The fluoridation of drinking water, which has been shown to prevent tooth decay. While you may be able to get bottled water delivered to your home with fluoride, it is so much easier to get it straight from your tap. Find out if your state fluoridates its water—not all states do—www.cdc.gov/fluoridation/statistics/2008stats.htm.

8

DOES EATING EGGS GIVE ME HIGH CHOLESTEROL?

I like to joke that eggs are the Rodney Dangerfield of food. They get no respect. In the last few decades, eggs have ping-ponged between being the darlings and the demons of the diet world. In their heyday, covered with cheese and nestled next to bacon and sausages, they screamed, "Guess who's on the Atkins Diet?" A few years passed and low-fat diets became the rage. Eggs were suddenly banished. There was a concern that eating eggs, even moderately, was responsible for high cholesterol levels, increasing the risk of heart disease. Now eggs are fighting their way back, trying to get the acceptance they deserve as one of the most nutritious and economical protein sources. In the process, they've left a lot of people confused about whether they should or shouldn't eat them.

I do like eggs, but there's more to address in this question than simply the benefits of eating or not eating them. It bothers me that eggs became the poster child for "bad" food simply because they contained cholesterol. As it turns out, for most people, cholesterol in a single food has a negligible effect on cholesterol levels in your blood. Cholesterol is naturally produced by your body. It is needed to make parts of cells and hormones, as well as to absorb certain vitamins. Your cholesterol level is the result of several factors: How much you eat, how much your body makes on its own, and how quickly your body clears it from your system. All of these play a role, as do your genetics, your weight, and your activity level.

Foods with cholesterol, if eaten in moderation, are an acceptable part of a healthy diet. Each egg contains around 185 mg of cholesterol. Most people can consume 300 mg per day and maintain normal blood cholesterol levels. If you are at high-risk for heart disease, drop that down to 200 mg per day. If you are one of the rare people who are very sensitive to dietary cholesterol, a so-called hyperresponder, you may need to carefully watch any dietary cholesterol.

Some fad diet book is always trying to convince you that it has the secret to good health, and it often involves totally cutting out a major food group. Sorry, but I just don't buy elimination diets. Eggs are a cheap, nutrient-dense protein source. One egg is only about 70 calories, with 6 grams of protein and only 1.5 grams of saturated fat. Eggs contain essential amino acids, vitamins, and folic acid. They provide choline, an important nutrient that helps regulate the brain, nervous system, and cardiovascular system. They also have a high carotenoid content, which is good for your vision.

Eggs seem to me like a pretty healthy addition to a diet. But like all animal protein, they should be eaten in moderation.

DR. B'S BOTTOM LINE:

Don't be swayed by fad diets that suddenly vilify foods that have been mainstays of our diets for centuries. There are many foods that we should eat more of and some we should eat less of, for many reasons. Don't let anyone tell you that eggs can't be part of a healthy, balanced diet.

CONCERNED ABOUT CHOLESTEROL?

Consider these tips:

- One egg a day is a good limit (seven per week). Evidence suggests this level is safe.
- Make sure to include in your count the eggs that are in prepared foods, such as mayonnaise, egg noodles, and most desserts.
- If you are cholesterol-sensitive, skip the yolk. That's where the cholesterol is.

- Remember to limit trans fats and saturated fats. These are converted to cholesterol by your body.
- If you are diabetic, you might be more sensitive to cholesterol in food. Talk to your doctor.

9

DO I NEED TO WASH PREWASHED LETTUCE MIXES?

When I first went to the CDC, I did a two-year fellowship as a disease detective investigating outbreaks of diarrheal disease. I was the envy of all my friends. After all, who wouldn't want to study poop every single day? At work, we kept a list on the wall of the riskiest foods. After every outbreak we would add a new culprit to the list.

I remember watching my colleagues at lunch, wondering after their years implicating virtually every food, what they would eat? Was anything truly safe? I also wondered if my own dining habits would change. I love sushi and raw oysters, rare hamburgers and runny eggs—all definite food safety no-nos. One of my bosses took the truly safe approach. His lunch was boiled: Boiled chicken, boiled vegetables, boiled everything! Safe, yes, but enticing? No! I wasn't going to go that far and you don't have to, either.

I quickly realized there is risk in everything we eat. It was up to me to know the hazards as best as I could, to be able to make the right decisions for myself, and to give advice to others. Some advice was a no-brainer. There was the guy who called and asked me whether it was safe to eat the Thanksgiving turkey he had forgotten about in the trunk of his car. His boss had given it to him two weeks earlier. Easy decision. Pitch the bird.

I didn't banish my favorite foods from my diet, but I definitely learned to be more discerning when it came to choosing what I ate. I became more aware of how food was being prepared and where it came from, and I learned to judge when to play it safe and when to be more daring.

I am frequently questioned about packaged produce mixes that say they are "prewashed." After years of being told to wash fruits and vegetables, now we are being told we don't have to. It is confusing. Like you, I'm concerned about prewashed lettuce mixes. Are they safe or should I still wash them?

Face it, who doesn't love the convenience of these ready-to-eat salads? They are an easy way to put a meal together and get nutritious greens into your diet. According to the USDA, sales of fresh-cut lettuce and leafy greens have reached more than $3 billion annually and the demand shows no signs of slowing. But produce has inherent risks. When salad greens are cut during harvesting, the exposed surfaces become vulnerable to potential contaminants. As thousands of pounds of greens are combined, washed, and then bagged, a small amount of bacteria can spread to contaminate a large amount of the mix. The CDC reported that one-third of the major food-borne outbreaks in 2011 were associated with fresh produce. Although the FDA oversees 80 percent of food in America, performing seven thousand inspections a year, they only visit some food processors an average of once every decade. Not very reassuring.

When I first came to ABC, I went out to Salinas Valley, California, where 85 percent of all leafy greens are grown, to see how producers had responded to an outbreak of E. coli O157:H7 from contaminated spinach three years earlier. These bacteria can cause one of the nastiest food-borne diseases. It takes only a few organisms to make you sick, and an infection can knock out your kidneys. Though they never figured out how this outbreak occurred, the most likely theory was that groundwater used to irrigate the spinach had been contaminated by wastewater from nearby pigs and cattle. I visited the production facilities at Earthbound Farm and saw how they had improved their facility and added additional quality control steps by implementing additional testing for harmful bacteria. Across the industry, new voluntary standards had helped to create a buffer between cattle and salad fields. All were good steps toward safer products.

However, critics urge caution. Erik Olson of the Pew Research Group, during an interview with ABC News, raised concerns that the standards are voluntary and that no binding rules govern the industry. In 2010, *Consumer Reports* tested 208 containers of lettuce (both bags and clamshells). It did not find any bacteria linked to outbreaks, such as E. coli 0157:H7, listeria, or salmonella, but did find high levels of coliforms, bacteria that live in your intestines. The presence of these germs indicates some level of fecal contamination, possibly from irrigation water, runoff from livestock, poorly sanitized equipment in processing facilities, or from sick workers. There are no established limits for these organisms in produce, but they're viewed as a rough guide to possible danger. While this sounds very alarming, the reality is that even an additional rinsing at home won't remove all these bacteria. Some bacteria are actually inside the leaves themselves. Even more, it is likely that your kitchen, or even your hands, may harbor bacteria that could contaminate the produce during additional rinsing. How clean is your sink, really?

Just as I learned to make my own informed choices, you need to gauge your own risk tolerance. The percentage of illness caused by lettuce mixes is small, but you might feel better buying heads of lettuce and making your own mix, although this does not remove all risk, either. If you do choose to use prepared lettuce mixes (and I do!), there are some things you can do to make it safer. Bacteria take time to grow and most grow faster at room temperature, so try to buy the freshest, coldest greens you can find. The *Consumer Reports* study found the lowest bacteria levels in packages more than five days from their "sell by" date. So *always* check that date and try to use the greens within a day or two of purchase. Before buying or using the mix, check to make sure there are no slimy, damaged, or bruised pieces. These are more vulnerable to bacteria. Proper storage is also critical. Make sure the package is well refrigerated at the market and refrigerate it as soon as you get home. I like to reach into the back of the store's refrigerator to get the package that is coldest. Keep it well sealed and away from raw meat or chicken, which could cross-contaminate it. I've looked into a lot of refrigerators and can't tell you how many times I've seen the greens sitting right underneath the package of chicken. Not a good idea.

DR. B'S BOTTOM LINE:

Serious outbreaks of illness associated with fresh produce have a lot of people concerned and confused about boxed and bagged greens and other vegetables. If you buy from a major supplier of prewashed, prepackaged greens and handle them properly, you may actually increase your risk by doing your own washing.

10

SHOULD I RINSE CHICKEN BEFORE COOKING IT?

When it comes to food safety practices in our own kitchens, sometimes we need to embrace actions to keep us safe that might seem counterintuitive. My friend Jodi would *never* think of cooking chicken, or any meat, before giving it a good rinse to "get rid of the germs." She's not alone. Even though this practice seems to make sense, Jodi's actually doing more harm than good. Let me explain why.

One of my favorite segments on *Good Morning America* is called "Doc at the Door," in which I come to your home and offer health advice in your living room. One of my first visits was to a neighborhood in New Jersey to check out safe cooking practices, specifically the dangers of cross-contamination from cooking poultry. What Lisa, the homeowner, didn't know was that I had coated a chicken with Glo Germ, a fine powder that spreads like bacteria through contact but is invisible except under a black light. It spreads around the kitchen just like salmonella or campylobacter, two common chicken contaminates, would. I watched Lisa prepare the bird. Afterward we turned off the lights and checked her hands and the surrounding area to see where the Glo Germ had landed. It was incredible. The place lit up with specks and splatters of simulated bacteria.

According to the CDC, each year, one in six Americans (48 million people) gets sick by consuming contaminated foods or beverages. Three thousand die of food-borne diseases. That's a lot of people with nasty bugs. Together, salmonella and campylobacter cause almost two million cases of food-borne illness and more than four hundred deaths annually. Many people, like Jodi, are grossed out at the thought of not rinsing their chicken before cooking, but it actually does more harm than good. When water hits the chicken, the resulting spray can spread pathogens all over your kitchen, especially the area by your sink, cutting boards, and faucet. This can result in cross-contamination if the bacteria come in contact with food that is sitting out nearby. Additionally, as you move about your kitchen touching bacteria-covered surfaces and items, you can further contribute to its spread.

Contrary to popular belief, water does nothing to kill bacteria and other pathogens. It will reduce the number of germs on the surface of the bird, but the only way to ensure that your chicken is safe to eat is to cook it until it reaches an internal temperature of 165°F. Thankfully, most people don't like to eat rare chicken.

To further protect yourself, when preparing raw poultry, handle it as little as possible. Wash your hands with soap and water for twenty seconds after touching it, being sure to remove rings and to scrub around your nails. Wipe down the surrounding area with hot soapy water or a mixture of one gallon of hot water and one tablespoon of liquid bleach. Use paper towels to clean areas that your chicken came in contact with, or if using cloth towels, stick them in the washing machine when you are done. Use caution when cleaning your cutting board, too, making sure not to spray it too forcefully with water. To sanitize your plastic cutting board, your best bet is to run it through the dishwasher. For wood, use hot soapy water. Afterward, throw your wet sponge in your microwave for two minutes or in the dishwasher to sanitize.

DR. B'S BOTTOM LINE:

Food safety is, and should be, a major concern for cooks, but there is a lot of confusion about what to wash and what not to wash before cooking. When your concern is bacteria rather than dirt, use caution. The spray of water can actually spread germs instead of containing them.

EASY GUIDELINES FOR PREVENTING CROSS-CONTAMINATION IN YOUR HOME

- Refrigerate chicken, meat, and seafood promptly after shopping.
- Keep raw meat, poultry, and seafood separated from other foods in your shopping cart and in your refrigerator. Make sure the protein is well wrapped and isn't leaking from its package and dripping on anything below.
- Use one cutting board for produce and a separate one for raw meat, poultry, and seafood.
- Invest in a reliable instant-read meat thermometer. It is the best way to test for doneness. Don't overcook the bird thinking it will kill more bacteria; 165°F keeps it safe, but also leaves the bird juicy and tender.
- Don't put cooked food on a plate that previously held raw meat, poultry, or seafood.

11

DOES USING TOO MUCH SALT CAUSE HIGH BLOOD PRESSURE?

Confession time! I used to be a real salt lover. I would put it on everything, often before tasting my food. I'm not alone, and for good reason. I'll admit it: A little sprinkle of salt makes food taste better. The problem is, from french fries to popcorn to processed and prepared foods, you get a *bunch* of salt every day—way more than you need—before you even season your food. Public health officials are very concerned that this dependency on salt plays a part in promoting high blood pressure, heart disease, strokes, and kidney disease.

When we talk about table salt and health, we are really talking about sodium chloride, our main source of sodium. No one should consume more than 2,300 mg of sodium a day, about a teaspoon of table salt. The recommended daily intake of sodium for *most* people (children, adults over fifty, African-Americans, and anyone with a history of high blood pressure, diabetes, or kidney disease) is even less, just 1,500 mg. Yet, here's the reality. If you are like the average American, you consume more than 3,300 mg of sodium every day, more than twice what you should. Men consume even more sodium than women, due to their increased caloric intake. In general, the amount of sodium you eat goes up in proportion to the number of calories you take in, making overweight people at even greater risk.

Many studies have shown that the more salt you ingest, the higher your blood pressure rises. The good news is there are also important studies showing that when you cut back on salt, your blood pressure comes down. Given that nearly one-third of adults have high blood pressure, addressing salt intake is an important step in improving your health.

You may be thinking, "How could I possibly eat that much salt? I don't put a teaspoon of salt on my food." Well here is a little secret: You could go through an entire day without reaching for a salt shaker and still get way too much sodium. Here's why: According to the CDC, more than 75 percent of the sodium you consume is from processed foods and restaurant meals, making it more of a challenge to cut back.

The World Health Organization (WHO) and the CDC have launched campaigns to try to reduce salt intake. You may hear a bit of a debate around salt and health, much (but not all) put forward by the Salt Institute, an industry group promoting salt consumption. Some of these studies find a much smaller benefit from salt reduction in terms of blood pressure control. They feel that the jury is still out and that promoting salt reduction should wait for more definitive data. Now, I am no salt expert, but in this debate, I side with the world's public health authorities. From my read, the weight of the evidence suggests that, at least for a considerable portion of the American population who are at risk for high blood pressure or who already have it, there *is* a connection and cutting back on salt makes a lot of sense.

Here are some tips to reduce your salt intake:

- Read food labels. Sodium is listed on the nutrition facts. I know it's hard to always do, but try to keep track for a couple of days to figure out where your salt is coming from. Look at every label! Even things that don't taste salty, like soda, contain sodium.
- When you are eating at a restaurant, ask for low-salt options. Many restaurants have them. Also, take a look at the nutrition facts the next time you are at a fast-food restaurant, if they are available. In addition to tons of calories and fat, most fast food is loaded with sodium.
- When you are in the supermarket, stick to the aisles around the edges of the store—where the produce, refrigerated, and frozen foods are. Avoid the middle of the store where the processed foods are. By "shopping the perimeter" you will increase your intake of fruits and vegetables and decrease the temptation to buy less healthy foods. Your sodium intake will go way down.
- When buying processed foods, look for the low-salt or no-salt varieties. You can always add a little back.
- Experiment using other herbs and spices to give foods a little zing. In addition to doing something really good for your health, you may find you like the new flavors.

DR. B'S BOTTOM LINE:

The bulk of the evidence supports the idea that excess sodium does, in fact, raise your blood pressure. It also suggests that cutting back on salt reduces your blood pressure. But even if you don't believe that the connection between salt and high blood pressure exists, salty foods also tend to be less healthy foods. Skip salty, overly processed foods and you will also lower your risk of obesity and heart problems.

HOW MUCH SALT IS IN THAT?

A quick look around the supermarket found surprisingly high amounts of sodium in recommended single-serving sizes that were also surprising. (I don't know anyone who eats ⅙ of a frozen pizza and calls it a day!)

Food	Sodium
1 teaspoon Dijon mustard	120 mg
2 tablespoons Skippy Creamy peanut butter	150 mg
1 big Snyder's pretzel	240 mg
1.1 ounces original Goldfish	250 mg
½ cup canned Del Monte cut green beans	340 mg
2 tablespoons Wish-Bone Italian salad dressing	340 mg
9 Tater Tots	420 mg
½ cup Ragu Traditional pasta sauce	480 mg
1 cup Hamburger Helper Cheesburger Macaroni	760 mg
⅙ frozen DiGiorno Four Cheese pizza	850 mg
½ cup Campbell's Chicken Noodle soup (condensed)	890 mg

12

ARE MY SLEEP HABITS MAKING ME FAT?

As a doctor, I can talk about the importance of getting enough sleep until I sound like Charlie Brown's teacher, "wah, wah, wah." I can ramble on about how sleep deficits result in irritability, a decrease in cognitive function, and increased risk for heart disease and diabetes, and everyone says, "Yeah, yeah, okay." But when I say, "Not getting enough sleep can make you fat," suddenly ears perk up. Now that I have your attention, let's examine the importance of getting a good night's sleep.

Adults need between seven and eight hours of sleep a night; children need even more. Since the 1960s on average, adults have gone from about eight to nine hours of sleep per night to seven hours. Almost a third of adults get less than that. During that same time period the obesity rate has increased—a lot. A big question has to be, is there a connection? Does a lack of proper sleep lead to obesity or does obesity lead to a lack of proper sleep?

It turns out that both are likely true. First let's tackle the most intriguing part of that question, how insufficient sleep promotes weight gain. The current thinking focuses on two critical hormones in the regulation of appetite, leptin and ghrelin. On a simple level, leptin is secreted by fat cells and tells the brain that you are full: Time to stop eating. Ghrelin is secreted primarily by the stomach and stimulates appetite: Bring on the food. The interplay between these two hormones has a very important role in how much you eat and when you feel full.

Numerous studies have shown that when you are sleep-deprived, your level of leptin decreases, while your level of ghrelin—along with your appetite—increases. Not surprisingly, when sleep-deprived subjects were given open access to food they ate more. In addition, sleep deprivation can slow your metabolic rate. In other words, you are going to feel hungrier, burn fewer calories, and have more waking hours in which to eat. Put these factors together and they strongly suggest that lack of adequate sleep promotes weight gain.

Now let's look at the other side of the question: Does obesity lead to poor sleep? This one is easy. Obesity is a risk factor for snoring and obstructive sleep apnea, a sleep disorder in which your airway gets blocked off for periods of time while you sleep. The connection to obesity may be from increased fat being deposited around the airways, which causes them to narrow. People with obstructive sleep apnea toss and turn at night as they try to open these airways.

So what are you to do? My take is that you can't keep squeezing sleep time into whatever is left over after work and play. It needs to get the same respect and protection as these other time commitments. Clearly it's easier said than done, but the development of good sleep habits is critical to good health. Oh, and did I mention that it may also help you lose weight?

DR. B'S BOTTOM LINE:

There are many reasons we need to get enough sleep. Your heart, brain, mood, and waistline will thank you. Pick whichever one motivates you and make an effort to develop good sleep practices. The key to good sleep is developing a routine that sets you up to succeed and sticking to it every night. Here are a few tips: Try not to exercise, eat a heavy meal, or drink alcohol close to bedtime.

13

CAN DRINKING DIET SODA MAKE ME GAIN WEIGHT?

Pet peeve alert! I can't tell you how many times I have to hold my tongue when I see someone order a double cheeseburger, large fries, onion rings, and . . . a diet soda. While I'd rather they order the diet soda over a can of regular cola, I really wish they ordered a regular-sized burger, a side salad, and a glass of sparkling water. That's just me.

Many public health leaders lay a lot of the blame for our current epidemic of obesity on sugary beverage consumption. I am one of them. But what about diet drinks? As obesity rates have risen, so has our appetite for artificially sweetened beverages. Is there a relationship? There have been headline-grabbing studies linking diet soda consumption to weight gain and a higher risk of obesity and associated illnesses including strokes, heart attacks, and diabetes. How could drinking a no-calorie beverage possibly be harmful?

If you normally drink two to three cans of soda a day and switch to diet soda, with everything else remaining the same, you would lose between thirty and forty pounds over the course of a year. So why are so many diet soda drinkers not losing weight? There are two main avenues of research to explain this: One focused on biology, the other on behavior.

The biologic research revolves around the soda drinker's dependence on sweetened foods. Using artificial sweeteners, which are hundreds to thousands of times sweeter than natural sugar, can lead to a phenomenon known as "taste distortion." Essentially, the "set point" for sweetness in the brain is altered, leading to increased consumption of sugar calories in other areas of the diet. You simply crave more sweet stuff. Other research suggests that sweetened beverages may trigger hunger and increased food intake by only partially satiating the body's desire for high-sugar foods. Some studies suggest that these sweeteners can actually lead to a spike in blood levels of insulin, which would in turn lead to food cravings.

Then there is the behavioral research that explores why we make our dietary choices. For example, there seems to be a misguided notion among many diners that ordering a diet soft drink gives them permission to splurge a bit more since they are "saving all those calories." They may overestimate how many calories they are cutting and instead overcompensate in other areas of their diet.

In the scientific community the connection between artificially sweetened beverages and weight gain is not universally accepted. Could diet sodas be tricking our brains into craving additional sweetness from our foods? Could they be spiking our insulin, which in turn leads us to consume additional calories? All of these things are possibilities. However, the existing research has yet to peg this down as fact. For now we have the simple fact that swapping zero-calorie drinks for sugar-laden beverages does reduce total caloric intake, as long as all else remains equal. In light of this, I will still recommend diet soda as a better alternative to sugary drinks for those who must have sweetened beverages.

DR. B'S BOTTOM LINE:

There's a lot of research out there, but right now it's inconclusive. While diet soda might not make you gain weight, consuming sodas, even diet sodas, adds no nutritional value to your diet. Try swapping in good, old-fashioned water for that soda. You'll get your hydration, and it's a completely natural beverage to boot!

GOOD-BYE SODA, HELLO SAVINGS

Just think of how much money you would save over the course of a year if you gave up your two (or more) cans of soda a day habit. You would save more than $250. Multiply that by the number of people in your family who drink soda and the savings are dramatic. I suggest investing in a seltzer maker, a machine that carbonates your water. That's what I did. You can have carbonated water whenever, with no lugging cans and bottles from the supermarket. Add a splash of lemon or lime if you like a tart drink or a splash of orange or cranberry juice for something sweeter.

14

DO MOST COLLEGE FRESHMEN GAIN FIFTEEN POUNDS?

The term "freshman fifteen" has become part of our lexicon. We were talking about freshman weight gain when I went to college, and my patients and their parents talk about it to me now. I took it for granted that there must be some validity to it. Think about it. Dining in college is a teenager's dream: All-you-can-eat buffets loaded with burgers, pizza, and soft-serve ice cream. Yes, there are healthy choices as well. But let's get serious. Few adults would choose such offerings; how could teens?

But does this lead to double-digit gains? That is a lot of weight. I decided to check it out for myself and headed back to college for *Good Morning America* for my "Doc at the Dorm" segment. I grabbed my backpack, threw on my sweatshirt, and headed to Boston University to see how freshmen were faring in the dining halls. What I saw wasn't pretty. For lunch, one petite woman had pizza, two servings of pasta, chicken, broccoli, and ice cream for a total of almost two thousand calories! That's about what she should be eating in an entire day. She wasn't alone. I watched the whole table take multiple trips to the dining line, often four and five go-rounds.

A couple of years ago the Department of Agriculture came out with new food guidelines. They threw out the food pyramid and went with a much easier tool for remembering how to balance your diet, the Food Plate. Basically you should divide your plate into quarters. Half should be fruits and vegetables, a quarter lean protein, and a quarter whole grains. How hard could that be? The plates I saw on campus? Not even close! I wouldn't know how to begin to classify some of these meals.

College is a big transition, with new freedoms and responsibilities. At home, kids are rarely treated to a smorgasbord at every single meal. At college, there is no parent intoning, "I think you've had enough." And those extra calories don't just come from the cafeteria. With a twelve-ounce cup of beer averaging one hundred and fifty calories, drinking adds more calories.

But freshmen are active as well, right? That's what I thought, until I visited the gym and took a look around. Where were the freshmen? The ones I talked to in the dining hall admitted they weren't working out. For many, the increased workload in college and all the transitions made it difficult to find the time for exercise. Everyone *planned* to get started working out soon, but "soon" kept getting pushed back. I began to wonder if the "freshman fifteen" was actually an understatement.

After some investigation, I found my fears unwarranted. There have been many studies that look at weight gain during freshman year. Guess what they found? In 2009, a review of twenty-four published studies found that on average, freshmen gain just under four pounds, nowhere near the fifteen pounds we expect. This is a bit more than the typical noncollege teen but not by much. The term "freshman fifteen" wasn't even coined until it appeared in *Seventeen* magazine in 1989, with no data to support that number. It was taken as gospel and has spread ever since.

While the overstatement of weight gain should give high school seniors some peace of mind, they shouldn't discount the potential weight gain that could await them. Learning to eat well in a college cafeteria is hard for many who don't have the tools to make good choices. The best way to prevent unhealthy adults is to provide a good framework for our kids long before they go to college. Teach your kids about portion control. We shouldn't expect our kids to skip french fries entirely, but we can let them know they shouldn't eat them every day. If they splurge at one meal, they should learn to compensate with lighter fare the next one. It's not just book knowledge that they should gain while living away. They need to be preparing for their lives as independent adults. Taking care of their health is a big part of that.

Another reality is that many people, especially boys, continue to grow during their college years and some weight gain is appropriate. I'm a shining example of this. I just kept on growing until I was twenty-two. When I go back to my high school reunions, I am always asked why I didn't play on the basketball team. I remind them, I wasn't six foot six in high school.

While we can celebrate the overstatement of the "freshman fifteen," we shouldn't get too excited. Many people experience a moderate but steady weight gain, typically through the five years after college. These yearly increases are when pounds really can add up. Once kids stop growing, leave school, and get jobs, their lives become more sedentary, which makes it much easier to gain weight. It's even more critical that young adults maintain good eating habits as they make that transition to "the real world."

DR. B'S BOTTOM LINE:

The "freshman fifteen" is a fake! However, show your kids how to eat healthfully and they'll avoid the slow but steady weight gain that starts during college years and continues afterward. The earlier you teach your kids about the importance of a balanced diet and physical activity, the more you set them up for a healthier and longer life.

2

ON YOUR MARK, GET SET, MOVE!

*Your Questions on Exercise, Fitness,
and Sports Performance*

Like changing your diet, when it comes to exercising, it's all about getting started by doing something.

As with many things in life, we have a tendency to overthink exercise. You don't need to run a 10K or complete a triathlon to be healthy. You just need to move. Every day you have opportunities to be a little more active than you are. You can park farther from your destination. You can take the stairs instead of the escalator. You can get up and go for a walk instead of eating lunch at your desk.

It's easy to talk yourself out of exercising for all the wrong reasons. You might think you need to exercise at a certain time of the day for it to really "count." You might think you need to exercise for a certain amount of time to get benefit. You're tired. You're hungry. The list goes on.

As much as you might be tempted to take the lazy route, don't. Physical activity is one of the most important things you can do to keep healthy. It's one of the best ways to lower your risk of cardiovascular diseases, type 2 diabetes, and even some types of cancers. It helps control high blood pressure and high cholesterol and is critical for maintaining and losing weight.

Physical activity also builds muscle, which burns more calories and also prevents fractures as you age. It gives you more energy and less stress. It can even help you sleep better and improve your sex life. What's not to like?

If you are a people person, join a group activity to keep you motivated, or engage a nearby exercise buddy to keep you accountable. If you enjoy more solitary time, download a book or some music on your iPod and off you go.

Luckily, being active doesn't mean you'll have to spend a lot of money or a lot of time, as you will learn. You don't need to join a fancy gym to work out. There are exercise videos and online programs that cost virtually nothing. I love to hop on my bike and go for a ride with my kids whenever the weather cooperates. My wife goes for power walks with her friends or jogs in the neighborhood to save the time she would spend traveling to the gym. A friend of mine swears by her subscription to YogaGlo, which streams yoga classes. When she's out of town or short on time, she follows a class on her iPad.

Here's the truth. No matter how you do it, just do something. Make it a way of life. You and a pair of sneakers—the beginning of a beautiful relationship.

15

CAN I BE FAT AND FIT?

In 2006 I made a trip to Jackson, Mississippi, to speak at a public health summit on preparing for a bird flu pandemic. However, my memories of that trip have nothing to do with flu; they have to do with what I had for lunch.

Let me explain. Mississippi is the fattest state in the country. More than a third of all Mississippians are obese; another third are overweight. The governor at the time, Haley Barbour, looked the part: big-jowled and big-bellied. Governor Barbour spoke at the summit, exhorting people to prepare for the flu, and then invited me and a few other health leaders up to his office for lunch. In his conference room we sat down to quite a spread: Each plate was loaded with a big heap of mashed potatoes smothered in gravy, a couple of pork chops, and a side salad. We passed around a large gravy boat full of ranch salad dressing. Governor Barbour was one of the first to receive it, sitting at the head of the table with his wife, Marsha, at his side. He started to ladle the dressing onto his salad. I could see Marsha watching him closely, a bit of a concerned look on her face. After about the third spoonful, Marsha grabbed his hand and said something like, "Haley, that's enough!" The governor gave us a big smile and said, "You know, have you seen Governor Huckabee? Did you see how much weight he lost? I don't like that at all! I like Governor Richardson. He and I like to eat. We're what you call fat but fit." We all gave a big chuckle and carried on with our meal but the image has stuck with me all these years. The governor of the fattest state in America sitting down to discuss public health problems while chowing down on pork chops. It was like something out of Dickens.

Surprisingly, this is a question I've been asked a lot: Can you be fat and fit? Was the governor on to something? Could he justify those extra pounds by implying he had athletic ability or was still otherwise healthy?

First, let's talk a bit about what it means to be fat. You can't just measure it in numbers of pounds, since that weight can be distributed on a short frame, a tall frame, or anything in between. There is always debate about what is the best measurement of "fatness," but physicians commonly use something called the body mass index (BMI). It is by no means perfect, but as long as you understand the limitations, it works quite well. It is calculated from your height and weight, and there are many calculators available online to help you compute your own. A normal adult BMI is 18.5–24.9; overweight is 25.0–29.9; and obese is 30.0 and above. For most people, your goal should be a BMI less than 25.

Let's get back to the governor's comment. Can fat people be fit? It depends somewhat on how you define fit. Fitness and health are not synonymous. When medical people talk about fitness, we are really talking about your heart: How well does it work to meet your body's needs? How much exercise can you handle? When the general public talks about being fit, it is often meant to encompass more: Being healthy and leading an active life.

Clearly you can be obese and not have medical problems. While obesity raises your *risk* for developing heart disease, diabetes, and orthopedic issues, not all people develop them. But it is kind of like asking: If you smoke cigarettes will you get lung cancer and emphysema? The answer is not necessarily—but your risk goes way up.

Numerous studies have also shown that there are obese people who have great exercise tolerance and strong hearts. There is good news for them. Obese people who are fit are at lower risk of numerous health problems than obese people who are not fit. Exercise, even if it doesn't lead to weight loss, does lead to health improvements.

Hopefully this will encourage everyone to exercise. Oh, and those of you who are at the right weight for your height but don't exercise? You aren't off the hook. Fitness matters for you, too.

DR. B'S BOTTOM LINE:

While it is possible to be fat and fit, most people who are fat aren't fit (and most people who are fit, aren't fat). The exercising you do to achieve fitness is good for your health and weight. If you are not at your ideal BMI, the efforts you make to move in the right direction can have big payoffs in terms of the quality and length of your life.

FIT FACT

Highly trained athletes will actually have high BMIs that would put them into the obese range due to their increase in muscle mass. But look, if you are a highly trained athlete, you don't need a number to tell you that you are fit.

16

SHOULD I PUSH MYSELF WHEN EXERCISING— NO PAIN, NO GAIN?

Have you ever taken a Spinning class? I have taken a total of two. That's it. And I only took the second one because I had to as part of a story I was doing for *Good Morning America* called "Doc at the Gym." I remember my first one like it was yesterday, standing up on this little bicycle, music pounding in my ears, the instructor forcing me to turn up the resistance and pedal faster and faster. I wondered whether my heart could actually burst through my chest wall. While my wife loved it, Spinning was way too intense for me. I quickly went back to a stationary exercise bike where I could control my own level of resistance and work hard, but still be able to read the newspaper.

Exercise has gone type A. Over the last few decades, workouts have been pushed to extremes. If you are from my generation, you'll remember the advent of the aerobic video, compliments of Jane Fonda and some others. While doing her donkey kicks, Fonda would purr in encouragement, "Feel the burn," fostering the "no pain, no gain" mentality. Today, rather than daily mile runs and aerobics classes, everyone seems to be running marathons and doing power yoga. We've established an exercise culture that implies physical activity doesn't count unless you push yourself beyond normal levels of exertion.

But does exercise really have to be a form of self-imposed torture? Regular exercise is one of the best things you can do for your health, but you need to remember you are asking your body to deliver more than usual. Your heart is working harder, beating faster as it pumps blood to your muscles. Your breath quickens as your lungs fill with air, oxygenating your blood. Your muscles and joints are working against increased resistance. The higher the intensity of the exercise, the harder your body has to work.

When it comes to pain, there are different sensations you can experience when exercising. Some are warning signs that must be heeded immediately;

others are just a normal part of challenging your body. Never exercise through chest pain or pain that radiates from your chest to your arms. This could be a sign that your heart is being overstressed. Stop what you are doing and call your doctor. While it is normal to feel a little uncomfortable and fatigued during exercise and after, it is another thing to feel extreme discomfort. If you feel sharp pain or light-headedness, you are asking too much of your body and you should immediately ease off. Either stop completely or back off and see if the pain resolves. This applies to any exercise: Weight lifting, aerobics, and even stretching. Acute pain means that something is wrong and could result in damage to your muscles, ligaments, or joints. Never try to just push through this kind of pain. Most trainers and instructors will give modifications during classes or sessions to lessen the intensity. There is no shame in adapting your practice to keep your body safe.

You may also feel burning in your muscles during intense exercise. This is due to a buildup of lactic acid, which is how your muscles respond to increased demand. It isn't dangerous, but you will find that it's harder to exercise for long periods of time once that "burn" sets in. Typically, the more fit you are, the longer you can work out without feeling this sensation.

In addition to feeling fatigue during exercise, it is normal to have a little discomfort for the next day or so when you have increased the intensity or used a new muscle group during your workout. Everyone knows what it's like on that first spring day when you hop on your bike, do yard work, or hit the tennis courts after months off. Ouch! As hard as it may be to go slow, it's best to try to ease into new activities gradually. Every summer I head to the beach where a good friend teaches step aerobics. For that one week I'm a "stepper" and boy, do I feel it the next few days. This is known as delayed onset muscle soreness, and it is thought to be a result of your body working to heal microscopic damage or tears to muscle fibers. As your body adapts to the new workout, your muscles will become stronger. In the meantime, anti-inflammatory pain relievers (like ibuprofen) or gentle massage can ease the symptoms. If possible, try to continue with light activity while your body recovers.

There are a number of ways to measure the intensity of your exercise routine. You can do it based on your heart rate, calculating how close you are to your maximal heart rate during exercise. A simple way to calculate your maximal heart rate is to subtract your age from 220. For moderate levels of exercise, shoot for a heart rate that is 50–70 percent of your maximal heart rate. For high-intensity activity, shoot for a target heart rate that is 70–85 percent of your maximal rate. You can also determine what is called your "perceived rate of exertion," using one of the available scales. What I think works best is even simpler. It is the simple talk test: If you can sing while you are exercising, you are working at a light level; if you can talk easily but can't sing, you are working at a moderate level; and if you can only say a few words before needing to take a breath, you are exercising at high intensity.

DR. B'S BOTTOM LINE:

When it comes to exercise, think "use it or lose it" rather than "no pain, no gain." Listen to your body. You can get all of the benefits of exercise if you get your heart rate up. There's no need to go for the burn or overdo it. If you experience sharp or continual pain during exercise, stop. Pushing through intense discomfort can do long-term or permanent damage.

TIPS FOR STARTING A NEW EXERCISE PROGRAM

- For new exercisers, consult a doctor before starting a workout program, to make sure you don't have any health conditions that could affect it.
- Find an activity you really like. You are much more likely to stick to it if you enjoy it. My wife likes Spinning classes, but I prefer the stationary bike. Try several things to see what works for you.

- Always start gradually and as your body becomes stronger, add to the time and intensity of your workout. Start with walking and then add jogging intervals if you feel up to it. You want to set yourself up for success, so it's important to stay injury-free.
- Mix up your workouts, not just to keep it interesting, but also to give your muscles time to recover. Have hard and easy days. Try yoga one day and an aerobics class the next.
- If you are new to the gym ask for an orientation to teach you how to properly use the machines. Many gyms offer a free session or two with a personal trainer as a joining incentive. Don't be shy about taking advantage of this (or asking for it if they don't offer). It's important to make sure you are starting with the proper weights and repetitions.
- Become familiar with your "perceived rate of exertion" and use that as a guide to make sure you are getting your heart rate up, but not overdoing it.
- If you do experience pain that persists or becomes worse, consult your doctor.

17

IF I'M EXERCISING, SHOULD I DRINK SPORTS DRINKS?

Be honest, aren't the sports drink ads great? Muscles flexing, bodies sweating, teams winning, athletes gritting their teeth and raising their arms in victory. If you want to play like the pros and look like the pros, drink the stuff they do, right? Actually, wrong. Of course, with about $3.9 billion in sales, it's no wonder you'd think otherwise. Unless you are exerting yourself as hard and as long as the pros do, you don't need sports drinks. Water works perfectly.

Sports drinks aggressively market themselves as being designed to provide rehydration and energy with a combination of water, carbohydrates (essentially sugar or high-fructose corn syrup), and electrolytes (essentially salts), intended to replenish what is lost through perspiration during exercise. But for most people, you get plenty of carbohydrates and salt through what you eat, making little need for replacement through what you drink. You have enough energy stored up in your body that can fuel your workouts. All you need is water and your body provides the rest.

So what's the downside with these beverages? Sports drinks taste better than water and are what the serious athletes use, right? Well, plenty is wrong with them. A typical twenty-ounce sports drink contains around 8 teaspoons of sugar, 275 mg of sodium, and 125 calories. If you are exercising to help control your weight or blood pressure, the last thing you need is unnecessary calories and salt. For every bottle of sports drink you consume, you need to run an extra mile just to stay in calorie balance.

The American Academy of Pediatrics recommends no sports drinks for children unless they are exercising vigorously (rarely seen in baseball!) for prolonged periods of time. The National Federation of State High School Associations recommends water as the best form of hydration, except for athletes undergoing intense activity for more than forty-five minutes or in settings of heat stress. For adults the same rules should apply. If you are playing like the pros, by all means, hydrate like them. For the rest of us, go for the water.

Hydration before, during, and after exercise is crucially important. Your body, *especially* in warm weather, needs to replace lost fluids. The experts are in agreement here. The best way to prevent dehydration is to drink *before* you are thirsty and continue to drink while exercising. So before heading out for a run or to the gym, drink water and then be sure to bring a container of it with you.

Oh, and make sure not to confuse sports drinks with energy drinks. They are two completely different things. Energy drinks contain substances that act as stimulants, such as caffeine or guarana. These are *not* to be used as exercise drinks.

DR. B'S BOTTOM LINE:

The obsession with sports drinks is a classic case of advertising trying to convince you to buy something you probably don't need. Water has done an amazing job providing rehydration for centuries. There is no evidence that for normal exercise any other supplement is needed. Save your money and the calories you just tried so hard to work off.

18

DO I NEED THIRTY MINUTES OF EXERCISE A DAY TO STAY HEALTHY?

If you read the recommendations, it's so easy to get discouraged. The U.S. Department of Health and Human Services recommends you get at least thirty minutes of exercise, five days a week, to see substantial health benefits. But let's get real. How many people can really commit to that? Not many. Well, there's some good news. Recent research shows that just half that amount of time can make a big difference to your health. That's really good news for those who find it hard to snag a half hour a day to work out and figure the bar is too high to even bother trying.

Here's the new finding. Researchers in Taiwan followed more than four hundred thousand adults over a twelve-year period. They were placed into one of five categories based on self-reported weekly exercise activity: Inactive, low, medium, high, or very high. The researchers calculated mortality risks and life expectancy for each group who exercised at all and compared them to those who admitted to doing absolutely nothing. The findings were very encouraging for people who don't exercise as much as is recommended. Just fifteen minutes of moderate exercise a day (or ninety-two minutes per week) was associated with a three-year increase in life expectancy and a 14 percent reduction in risk of death, compared with a sedentary lifestyle. With every additional fifteen minutes of exercise per day, participants further increased their life expectancy by 4 percent and reduced their risk of death during the study period. Does this definitively answer the question? Unfortunately not. They didn't randomly assign people to their level of exercise, people chose this on their own, so it's possible that people who chose to exercise more also made other decisions that contributed to the participants' improved health. But for me, I'm convinced that even small amounts of exercise can make a big difference to your health and longevity.

According to the CDC's most recent survey data, 33 percent of American adults *never* exercise and 55 percent don't consider themselves highly active. Inactivity increases with age, most likely due to increasing medical conditions that interfere with activity.

If you have a regular exercise regime of more than fifteen minutes, don't interpret this study as a message to cut back. Every additional increment showed benefit. But for those who don't do anything—try to work in fifteen minutes. It's not difficult. I promise! Just look to be more active in any way you can.

DR. B'S BOTTOM LINE:

Even fifteen minutes of exercise a day will improve your health and could possibly prolong your life. Don't be put off on the recommendations that tell you to do more. The most important thing is that you do something.

A FEW EASY TIPS FOR SNEAKING
IN EXTRA EXERCISE

- Climb the stairs instead of taking the escalator or elevator.
- Take your dog for an extra or longer walk.
- Park farther from the store when you do errands.
- If you ride the bus or subway, get off one or two stops early.
- When you find yourself just strolling, pick up the pace for added benefit.
- Do physical activity as a group to get everyone moving. There's more fun in numbers. Include family and friends on a bike ride, brisk walk, or hike. When exercise is done as a social activity, even non-exercisers seem willing to get moving.

- Volunteer for physical projects like Habitat for Humanity or gardening days at local schools or community centers.
- Most important, find something you like and start small. You are more likely to be successful and keep it going. You can always increase time and intensity later.

19

TO LOSE WEIGHT, IS EXERCISE MORE IMPORTANT THAN DIET?

We were having dinner with a good friend last week. I'll call him Dave. He was clearly annoyed. He had recently started a new exercise program with a trainer and hadn't lost a single pound. As he was talking, he scooped a second serving of french fries onto his plate. In that moment it all became a little clearer why his scale wasn't budging.

If you are trying to lose weight and it isn't working, there are usually two problems: You're eating more than you need and you are exercising less than you should. Weight loss is really pretty simple mathematics.

Everything you do burns calories, even watching television, sleeping, and reading this book. The more vigorous the activity, whether that be gardening, house cleaning, jogging, or playing sports, the more calories you will expend. If Dave kept working out and ate the same or less, he would lose weight. However, many studies show that when it comes to weight loss, what you put in your mouth matters a lot more than what you do at the gym.

To lose one pound you need to expend 3,500 more calories than you consume. In general, a safe, sustainable weight loss goal is no more than one to two pounds a week. If you divide that by seven days, you are looking at shifting your daily balance by 500 to 1,000 calories. However, you don't have to burn up that many calories per day, nor do you have to reduce what you eat by that many. Think about doing a combination of the two. For example, if you reduce your caloric intake by three hundred calories a day (basically a bit more than one large soda) and increase your activities to burn two hundred extra calories per day, you can expect a steady weight loss of approximately one pound per week.

So why isn't Dave losing weight? Let's examine some of the pitfalls that might be plaguing him. As a relatively new exerciser, his regimen is still building. Let's say over the course of an hour he is getting moderate exercise by lifting weights and using a treadmill. Over the course of an hour, he will burn three hundred to four hundred calories. However, since this is a big increase in activity, he may be tired and sit around more than usual during the rest of the day burning fewer calories than usual. So over the course of the day his total increase in energy isn't quite so high.

While some exercisers find their appetites decrease after working out, for others the opposite is true. For those looking to lose weight, there's nothing more sabotaging than feeling intense hunger after working out, especially when you are programmed to be rewarded with food for your efforts. Sometimes it's just thirst that gets the better of you. After a workout, instead of hydrating with a big glass of water, some exercisers will go for a calorie-laden drink from the club's snack bar and chow down on protein bars, forgetting they may contain more calories than what they just worked so hard to burn off. I know—it's discouraging. And guess what a lot of people do when they are frustrated: They eat! Talk about a catch-22!

Dave clearly felt that by signing up with a trainer, he'd earned the right to eat a bit more, even though the reason he started exercising was to help him lose weight. However, if he stops by the coffee shop and grabs a piece of coffee cake (440 calories) or a latte (190 calories), the weight loss value of his workout would be gone. He doesn't lose the benefits in terms of cardiovascular health, but he will be sorely disappointed when he steps on the scale.

Before you give up on adding aerobic exercise to your life purely for weight loss, remember that there are a lot of reasons to exercise in addition to losing pounds. It gets your heart pumping, which decreases your risk of cardiovascular diseases. It boosts your good cholesterol and decreases unhealthy fats called triglycerides. It makes you feel better mentally and emotionally by stimulating endorphins and other brain chemicals. It also releases stress and boosts your energy. Strength training builds muscle and muscle burns more calories than fat—so even when resting, you will burn more calories.

Remember, everything burns calories. You don't need to go to the gym to get fit. Every little thing adds up.

DR. B'S BOTTOM LINE:

The most important factor in losing weight is cutting back on how much you eat. It really is pretty hard to lose weight just by exercising, but that doesn't mean that exercise isn't important. Lifestyle changes that incorporate exercise with dietary changes are more successful than diet changes alone. Even more importantly, exercise has so many health benefits that have nothing to do with your waistline.

20

IS MORNING THE BEST TIME TO EXERCISE?

People ask me all the time: When is the best time of day to exercise? Behind this question lies a belief that there is an optimal time to work out, one in which the body gets better results with the same amount of effort. However, I don't buy into that. My answer is simple. The best time to exercise is the one that works best in your life so that you can stick to it. While there are some data to show that your strength and endurance are best later in the afternoon, the differences are not significant and shouldn't drive your exercise decisions. What really matters is that you incorporate physical activity into your day.

I am a morning person. Much to the chagrin of those in my family who like to ease into their day, I roll out of bed ready to go. That's why exercising first thing in the morning, before going to work, is best for me. It gives me energy and clears my head, so that once I hit my office I'm ready to go. I feel great during the day knowing that I've got my workout under my belt and don't have it hanging over me when things get crazy. Once I'm at my desk, I never know when I'll be able to slow down or finish the day, so postponing exercising would be very risky for me. Additionally, by the time I leave the office, I'm exhausted and ready for dinner and time with my family. Having to hit the gym in that condition is impossible. But that's just me. Many people I work with view their noon Spinning classes as a way to break up their day and burn pent-up energy. Others make a nighttime gym visit their evening social event because they don't like working out under time constraints. Most consistent exercisers have found their time and honor that commitment.

If you are new to exercise, don't overthink it. Pick a time to exercise that fits best with your lifestyle and schedule, the time that is hardest for you to make excuses for skipping. Start small and experience success first. A fifteen-minute power walk is a wonderful thing for your health and is so much easier to stick to than training for a marathon. Often if you are overly ambitious you can quickly burn out. Every January I see the same phenomenon: The gym I belong to gets crowded. Sometimes I have to wait to get on my favorite exercise bicycle or to use certain machines. The floor mats where I stretch out are wall-to-wall people. But I keep my calm; I know that by the first week in February things will be back to normal.

A survey by the Gallup organization found that only a quarter of all Americans get thirty minutes of exercise at least five times a week; slightly more than that don't exercise at all. Anything you can do to keep yourself out of the group that doesn't exercise at all is a really good thing. Don't get hung up on when the best time is for your body. Exercising in some way, at any time of day, is critical for good health.

DR. B'S BOTTOM LINE:

Find a time to exercise that works for you. You will be more likely to stay with it if it becomes a habit—whenever that time of day may be.

21

SHOULD I STRETCH BEFORE EXERCISING?

How many times have you driven by a park and seen runners in deep lunges, rhythmically bouncing as they stretch out before they take off around the track? Stretching has long been touted as the best way to prevent injuries and post-exercise soreness, but my wife swears in all her years of running, the only time she's been injured is during her pre-run stretching. It turns out she's not the only one. While it makes sense to warm up muscles before working out, stretching is not the best way to do it. Research shows that stretching does little to prevent injury during exercise and could actually *cause* muscle pulls or strains.

Now let me be clear: I'm not saying you shouldn't warm up before taking on intense exercise. A few years ago I did a nice job tearing my calf muscle by playing tennis without warming up. It took me out of the game for almost six months. I am now much more attentive to gently moving my muscles before I go all out. Here is the typical drill when I play tennis. My partner and I begin by lightly hitting the ball from the service line with a very soft half swing. We gradually work our way back to the baseline with first a soft and then a full swing. Those balls not hit right back to me, I let go at first. Then I'll do some gentle jogging to pick up stray balls. Slowly and gently my muscles warm up.

Whether it's tennis, running, or cycling, the safest way to warm up your muscles is to mimic the movements you will be doing, but at decreased intensity. Gradually increase your heart rate and get blood flowing to your muscles. As you start to feel warmed up you can increase your movements and build speed and intensity.

Numerous studies have looked at the issue of stretching and have found injury rates to be the same in those who did and did not stretch. A recent study involving the USA Track and Field Association looked at 2,700 runners. They found no difference in the injury rates of those who stretched before running and those who didn't. They did find that injuries were more common for heavier runners and those who had recently recovered from an injury. They also found that runners who were asked to switch their stretching routines as part of the study were more likely to get injured, implying the body adapts to routines. So if you are someone who swears by stretching before exercising, it may make sense to stay with it.

While stretching might not be recommended as a warm-up, it is important to work stretching into your daily life and exercise routine to build flexibility and balance, which are especially important as you age. Before you get out of bed, give yourself a few minutes to warm up, with very gentle movements, to get blood flowing. Gently pull your knees, one at a time, into your chest and give them a light hug to stretch your hamstrings. Slowly windshield-wiper your legs from side to side to loosen up your back. Tense your shoulders up and then shrug to relax them. Try to work a yoga or stretch class into your exercise regime. I took up yoga five years ago and find that the stretching I do helps with my posture and has reduced the strain on my back—but even in a class focused on stretching, we warm up first.

DR. B'S BOTTOM LINE:

Science strongly suggests that stretching before a workout does not prevent injuries or reduce post-exercise muscle soreness. A gentle and gradual warm-up is much better for your muscles.

22

WILL WEARING ION OR MAGNETIC JEWELRY IMPROVE MY SPORTS PERFORMANCE?

When my son, Jack, joined his travel baseball club he got a package of "team gear." Included was a bag with his team's logo, sunglasses, batting gloves, and surprisingly, an ion necklace. While all the kids whipped that necklace on with dreams of future major-league glory, Jack just put it back in the bag. I guess after living with me for so long, he was savvy enough to know that there was no connection between wearing that piece of jewelry and improving his baseball skills.

These manufacturers' websites make grandiose claims. According to one website, ionic necklaces "maximize performance by neutralizing the effects of positive ions in our environment." Doing so, they claim, can result in healing properties that promote well-being and balance, improve your immune system, even increase energy, power, focus, and sleep. Unfortunately, there's no scientific proof that this is true. Bracelets and necklaces do not generate negative ions. And even if they did, there is no science to suggest health or athletic benefits.

Use of these necklaces and bracelets isn't limited to baseball. They are also worn by star athletes who play basketball, golf, and football. They are seen on action heroes in the movies. Sadly, these endorsements encourage children and adults to spend a lot of money on something with no proven value.

Now, I have no problem with the player who carries a rabbit's foot or has an at-bat ritual of patting his head, pulling at his shirt, and kicking the plate four times. This kind of superstitious behavior may relax a player and clearly doesn't encourage people to waste their money mimicking it. But when you are paid to endorse a product that is worthless and is being marketed to the public, *that* bothers me. A lot.

In fact, for the last decade, the Federal Trade Commission, which regulates consumer fraud, has been going after makers of ionized jewelry for making false claims about their ability to relieve pain from arthritis and other chronic conditions. This happened in 2003 against the company that made Q-Ray bracelets when their advertising claimed that ion bracelets provided immediate pain relief through "enhancing the flow of bio-energy." The judge in the case said the defendants might as well have said: "Beneficent creatures from the 17th Dimension use this bracelet as a beacon to locate people who need pain relief, and whisk them off to their homeworld every night to provide help in ways unknown to our science." In a final ruling, the U.S. Court of Appeals upheld the initial court finding. The company returned almost $12 million to more than 248,000 consumers.

Magnet therapy is equally unfounded. Promoters claim wearing magnetic jewelry, or placing magnets around areas of the body, can relieve arthritis, headaches, and stress. Some go as far as saying it can heal broken bones, reverse degenerative diseases, and even cure cancer. However, the FDA's stance on magnets is clear. To date, the FDA has *not* approved of any magnets promoted to treat a medical condition or to affect the structure or function of the body. Because these devices do not have this clearance, they are in violation of the law, and are subject to regulatory action if they represent themselves as being approved for treatment of medical conditions.

If you are using these to treat a medical condition, be very careful. It might be tempting to try alternative therapies as a quick fix, or in the hope they will help what ails you, even if in only a metaphysical way. But there is the potential danger of delaying seeking traditional medical attention that is scientifically proven to be more valuable. If you want to supplement your medical care with an alternative approach, do so with open eyes and involve your doctor. I will often work with patients who want to try an alternative approach as long as it is safe. The problem I have is when a treatment supported solely by anecdote is held in the same regard as one that has been rigorously tested through clinical trials.

DR. B'S BOTTOM LINE:

Ionic and magnetic jewelry are great examples of unproven pseudoscience being used to make a lot of money for manufacturers who don't have your well-being at heart. Whenever you see medical claims for nontraditional therapies, talk to your doctor about them before spending your hard-earned dollars. It's one thing if you want to buy them just to have them. It's another if you are using them to replace proven remedies that might truly help you.

TOO GOOD TO BE TRUE?

There are several websites I like to turn to when I have questions as to whether something I've heard about is the real deal or too good to be true. Check out these for honest answers:

- National Center for Complementary and Alternative Medicine: Part of the National Institutes of Health, its mission is to thoroughly investigate the usefulness and safety of alternative approaches to health (www.nccam.nih.gov).
- Federal Trade Commission: Miracle Health Claims: Provides tips on how to avoid becoming a victim of health fraud (www.ftc.gov/bcp/edu/pubs /consumer/health/hea07.shtm).
- Quackwatch: Your Guide to Quackery, Health Fraud, and Intelligent Decisions: Provides information about health-related frauds, myths, fads, fallacies, and misconduct (www.quackwatch.com).

3

OH DOCTOR, ONE MORE THING!

Your Questions When I'm Walking Out the Door

For me, few things are more rewarding than the relationships I develop with the patients I treat. One of the best things about being a pediatrician is that I get to connect with people of all ages: Children, teens, young adults, their parents, and grandparents. When they visit, I don't just spend time on their physical exams. I spend more time exploring who they are and what they do. To be a good physician, I need to know about all aspects of my patients' lives: How is it going in school? What do they do in their free time? Do they have a best friend? How are things at home? Do they like to drink water? What do they eat for breakfast? Mostly, I want to know if they are making smart decisions about their health and to help them if they are not.

One of my favorite parts of the visit is near the very end, when I think we are just about finished. After we've talked and I've examined whatever needs examining, as I'm about to get up and head to the door, it happens—the out-the-door question. That is when my patients tell me why they really came to see me. Sometimes it is about something that has been really worrying them for a long time; at other times it is just something about which they have been curious. I sit back down, and we talk some more. That is when our relationship really deepens.

In this section I'll address many of these questions. These are things that you may think you know the answers to, but I'd be surprised if you knew the answers to them all. Hopefully you'll pick up some information that will help you make smarter health decisions, decisions based on the truth.

23

WILL COUNTING SHEEP CURE MY INSOMNIA?

When I wake up in the middle of the night and can't fall back to sleep because of something on my mind, what works best for me is to wake up my wife and let her know what's bothering me. After about five minutes of recounting my worries, I fall back to sleep like a baby. Unfortunately, I can't say the same for her. To save my marriage, I've learned to keep a pad by the bed, so when I awake with something I can't stop thinking about, I write it down. I then relax knowing I'll deal with it in the morning. It really works, and my wife gets much more sleep.

Insomnia is incredibly common, and there are two main types: Having trouble falling asleep and having trouble staying asleep. All who've experienced them would agree there's nothing more frustrating than not being able to sleep when you want to. According to the National Sleep Foundation, an industry organization, 65 percent of Americans report insomnia occasionally, while 44 percent of those respondents experience insomnia almost every night.

Although it is common, you should not ignore insomnia. New onset of insomnia can be a sign of many different health problems, including heart disease, asthma, obstructive sleep apnea, and depression. If you have persistent insomnia, keep a sleep diary and record when you go to bed and when you wake up, so you can discuss it with your doctor. You will rest better knowing that your problem doesn't go beyond just sleep difficulty.

Like me, many people who have sporadic trouble sleeping are thinking about something. I remember as a kid being told that counting sheep would help me fall asleep. Taking your mind off thoughts by practicing a monotonous drill designed to distract your brain seems to make sense. But as I began to research better sleep solutions, counting sheep was not found to be as successful as other methods.

Oxford University researchers did a study to determine which pre-sleep behaviors best encouraged sleep. They asked forty-one insomniacs to engage in one of three thought patterns before trying to sleep: To envision a peaceful scene, such as being on a quiet beach; to count sheep; or to engage in their usual pre-sleep routine. Those who concentrated on relaxing imagery fell asleep an average of twenty minutes earlier than sheep counters or those doing nothing. The researchers concluded that counting sheep was so repetitive that the brain looked for distractions and, in doing so, broke the relaxation cycle. Conversely, the thought of calming activities engaged enough brain power to keep subjects from reverting back to the worrisome thoughts and allowed them to relax. A later study at Oxford found that insomniacs tended to think of more unpleasant images at bedtime than people who had less difficulty falling asleep, further support for the benefits of visualizing pleasing settings.

In 1990, I was doing public health work in Bangladesh and took a vacation on Ko Samui, a beautiful island in the South China Sea off the coast of Thailand. I rented a little hut on the beach surrounded by palm trees. I still remember my daily routine of stretching out in a rope hammock between two of those trees and falling to sleep listening to the gentle surf on the shore. That is the image I think of when I'm having trouble falling to sleep. There are enough things going on to keep me interested and to block out the cares of the day. Think back over your life: Is there some place or image that means relaxation to you?

DR. B'S BOTTOM LINE:

To fall asleep faster, put the livestock out to pasture. Banish negative thoughts and visualize calming scenes. If you wake up with something on your mind, writing it down or telling someone what's worrying you can help you get back to the business of sleeping.

TIPS TO ESTABLISH A
SUCCESSFUL BEDTIME ROUTINE

Anyone who has been a parent knows the importance of routine in getting the little ones to bed. For some reason, this practice doesn't always translate to what we need to do for ourselves. All sleep experts say the same thing: The key to good sleep is routine.

- Go to bed and get up at the same time every day. There is more and more research supporting health benefits from consistent schedules.
- While exercise during the day helps with sleep, try not to do it too close to bedtime. That can actually make sleep more difficult.
- Pay attention to what you eat and drink before bedtime. Try to finish eating and drinking several hours before bedtime and avoid anything too filling, fatty, or spicy.
- Avoid caffeine, nicotine, and alcohol close to bedtime. Although alcohol can help you fall asleep, it can disturb your sleep later.
- Create a conducive sleep environment. I use eyeshades to block out excess light. My wife uses earplugs to block out my snoring! A good friend uses a white noise machine.
- Only use your bedroom for sleep and sex. Don't watch TV or play video games there.
- Park your electronics. Leave them in another room so you're not tempted to check your email if you wake in the middle of the night.
- If you don't fall asleep within thirty minutes, get up, go into another room, and read or relax until you feel sleepy.

24

CAN I MAKE UP FOR LACK OF SLEEP DURING THE WEEK BY SLEEPING LATE ON WEEKENDS?

I have two teenage sons who stay up way past my bedtime. When they have big school assignments I know they are up even later. In typical teenage fashion, on weekends they both sleep in, trying to compensate for those late nights. They aren't alone. Even I try to catch up on sleep on the weekends after a busy week. When there is a lot of medical news, I'm up at 5 a.m. for *Good Morning America,* and I'm not home until almost 8:30 p.m., after *World News.* The big question is this: Do those extra hours on the weekend make up for the weekday shortfall?

First, let's talk about why sleep matters. Most adults need seven to eight hours of sleep per night; less than that and you will probably feel sleepy during the day. The consequences of insufficient sleep actually go way beyond sleepiness. You can't function your best at work if you are tired. Specifically, sleep deprivation affects your ability to concentrate, attention to detail, error rates, manual dexterity, and creative thinking. If you do manual labor or operate equipment it can be dangerous. Fall asleep on the job and you may be looking for a new one.

Sleep is vital to many of our bodily functions. Everything from how our bodies fight infections to how we handle sugar depends on it. Inadequate sleep is also associated with an increased risk for diabetes, heart disease, obesity, and depression. While most of us would never get behind the wheel of a car drunk, almost 20 percent of serious car accidents involve sleepiness as a contributing factor. I still remember feeling myself nodding off at a red light after a thirty-six-hour shift as a pediatric resident. Scary.

According to the CDC, more than a third of U.S. adults report sleeping fewer than seven hours on average per night and the numbers are on the rise. The Institute of Medicine attributes the problem in large part to how we are living our lives: Longer workdays, more shift work, and then staying up later at night with our electronics: Television, video games, and the Internet.

So what about catch-up sleep? Can you skimp on sleep during the week and make up for it on the weekend? Scientists at Walter Reed Army Institute of Research set out to answer that very question. They divided sixty-six subjects into four groups, restricted their sleep to varying amounts of time (three, five, seven, or nine hours per night), and measured how well they performed on various tests of attention afterward. Then they let them all have three nights of recovery sleep (eight hours per night) to see if their performance would improve. Their findings? All of the groups performed worse than the group getting nine hours of sleep; in general the less sleep, the worse the performance. What about those nights with catch-up sleep? Well, performance improved but not up to their baseline. Unfortunately, saving your sleep for the weekend just doesn't get the job done.

There are other concerns about regularly trying to compensate by oversleeping on the weekends. Getting too much sleep on one day can make it harder to fall asleep that night, setting off another chain of sleep challenges. Your sleep-wake cycle is regulated by an internal circadian clock that sets your body's sleep and wake times. Maintaining regular waking and sleeping times helps regulate your bodily functions and is the best for your health. Playing with those patterns can have serious health consequences.

DR. B'S BOTTOM LINE:

Try to get at least seven hours of shut-eye each night. The best way to do this is by keeping a regular sleep schedule, even on the weekends, when it's tempting to sleep longer. And if your life just won't let you do this? Catch an extra hour whenever you can but realize it won't fully recharge your batteries.

25

IS OWNING A PET GOOD FOR MY HEALTH?

I'm a dog person; always have been. Right now we have two of the worst-behaved dogs ever, but like most pet owners, I couldn't dream of living without them. They greet me at the door, tails wagging, and provide unconditional love. And no matter how tired I am, they make me get off my butt to walk and play with them.

I come from a dog family. Growing up we always had at least one. Even after my siblings and I moved out, my parents had a succession of black Labs, until recently, when their latest, Hannah, passed away. This is the first time I can remember that they have been without a dog at their side.

I frequently have discussions with families about adding an animal into their lives. I help them to determine if it's the right time and if so, what type of pet would be best. I hadn't really thought much about whether getting a pet at my parents' age would be a good thing. They are in their early eighties and I know how much work a dog can be. Yet I have such positive memories of their interaction with their pets and know their dogs contributed to their well-being. I picture their long walks with Hannah, the companionship she provided to them, and how they loved when people would stop to stroke her and chat about how pretty she was. These activities and interactions enriched their lives, especially as they grew older and became empty-nesters. I became curious whether there were proven health benefits of owning pets, especially in the "golden years."

There have only been limited studies on this topic and research is inconclusive. Some show benefits and some do not. For many studies, it is hard to know whether health benefits that are seen in pet owners are due to owning the pet or whether there is something fundamentally different about people who decide to own pets. A recent review of the issue by Dr. Harold Herzog in *Current Directions in Psychological Science* concluded that at this point, physical and mental health benefits are unproven. I tend to agree with him.

There can be health risks from having a dog or cat. According to the CDC, each year there are almost 90,000 falls related to pets. These falls often result in broken bones, and those most at risk are the elderly, especially those older than seventy-five. The most common cause of falls is one of the health benefits: Walking the dog. That's not all. Each year dogs bite more than four million people. More than 300,000 of those victims go to the emergency room. In addition to injuries, pets can be the source of a wide array of infectious diseases, from cat scratch disease, worms, and Lyme disease to diarrheal illnesses and ringworm.

There can be tangible benefits in having a pet, though. Walking your dog is a great way to incorporate exercise into your daily routine, if you get your heart rate up. Like my parents, being out with your pet is one way to help you stay socially connected if you have a social dog. You know the saying—if you want to meet someone, get a puppy. Those types of interactions are good for your health. Studies have shown that people who have more social relationships tend to live longer and be happier than people who are more isolated. Here again, you need to have the right kind of dog, one that's as social as you are. For some people, the connections to their pets—whether dogs, cats, fish, or other companions—are as strong as or stronger than the connections to other people. Those bonds can have a positive effect on your mental health and happiness, too.

No matter what your age and stage in life, owning a pet is not something to enter into lightly. A pet is a long-term emotional and financial commitment. Before deciding to get a pet, you need to make an assessment of whether you are able to care for it. Choose an animal that is suited for your lifestyle and fits in with your family life. A cat is much easier to care for than a dog, and different dogs have varying energy levels. My parents wisely chose to adopt Hannah, a very mellow adult dog, and would do the same if they were to get another. Obviously getting a dog when you are at a more advanced age has more challenges because of your own longevity issues. Think about what would happen to the pet if you were no longer able to care for it. Inquire if there is a friend or family member who might be willing to adopt it.

DR. B'S BOTTOM LINE:

Living with a companion animal may offer some health benefits, increase lon-gevity, and foster a feeling of connectedness to another living creature, but it also poses some risk. Whether the benefits outweigh the risks depends upon your particular health, temperament, and living circumstances. The scientific jury is still out on this one. For now, your decision to own a pet should *not* be determined solely by your desire to live healthier or longer.

26

WILL EATING DINNER TOGETHER MAKE MY FAMILY HEALTHIER?

Emotional health and physical health are inseparable. Part of being healthy emotionally is developing strong connections with family and friends. But these days, maintaining and strengthening those connections is harder than ever. Nowhere is this more apparent than in our own homes. Family members are pulled in so many directions. One thing that I hold sacred in our house is sitting down to a family dinner every night when I'm not on *World News*. With crazy schedules it's a hard thing to do. Between work, after-school sports, extracurricular activities, and competing with places our kids might rather be, it's not something that just happens naturally. But we make it work because it matters. Consistently connecting with your family is one of the most important things you can do for your kids.

As a pediatrician, I stress this to my patients, their parents, and anyone else who will listen. The benefits of family dinners are manifold. In addition to helping you keep up with your children's and spouse's activities, it says to your family that you value spending time together. It's a great way to check in to see how your kids are doing in school, not just academically, but socially and emotionally as well.

For more than sixteen years, the National Center on Addiction and Substance Abuse (CASA) at Columbia University has surveyed thousands of teens and their parents, looking for factors that affect the likelihood of teen substance abuse. It found parental interaction at the dinner table to be one of the most successful tools to raise healthy, drug-free children. The more frequently children ate dinner with their parents, the less likely they were to smoke, drink, or use drugs—or hang out with kids who do. Teens whose families ate dinner together fewer than three times a week were twice as likely to have used tobacco, nearly twice as likely to have used alcohol, and one and a half times as likely to have used marijuana than those who ate together at least five times a week. CASA's report, "The Importance of Family Dinners VI," shows kids want that time together. Sixty percent of teens who have dinner with their parents fewer than five nights a week wish they could do it more often.

Now, I take this research with a grain of salt. It's possible that eating dinner as a family is more a marker of a family that values being together, rather than the cause of less risky behavior by kids. It is possible that parents who make time to sit down with their children for dinner also keep better tabs on their children at other times, spend more time talking to them, and have stronger relationships. But these findings also make common sense. Not only that, but their recommended changes in behavior won't cost you a penny.

For one hour, my wife and I make everyone, including ourselves, turn off electronically. We put down our phones, iPods, and PDAs, and turn off our computers, TVs, and DVDs. With technology overtaking our daily lives, the art of conversation is becoming a relic. Breaking bread with your family forces everyone to talk. Even if it's just chatting some days, other nights it might be something more meaningful.

I admit it. Sometimes one of my kids' initial response to "What happened today?" is "Nuthin'," but by the time I recount my activities and my wife hers, the kids are perking up, often interrupting each other to fill in the blanks of their days. I end up hearing about so much more than the "boring" response to "How was your day?" when I am out of town and check in by phone. By telling my kids all about my day, the good, the bad, and the ugly, they see that even adults have to deal with highs and lows and be resilient. My kids are surprised to see the same interpersonal conflicts they are experiencing manifest themselves decades later between adults. I also talk about my job in a positive way, to teach them an important lesson: When you find something you love to do, work doesn't really feel like work.

There are also other, more tangible benefits. Eating together has been shown to increase the amount of healthy food kids eat. Seeing me load my plate with veggies signals them to do the same. Children are less likely to be overweight if they eat with their families. Additionally, sharing meals can also alert you to potential eating disorders, especially with adolescent girls.

DR. B'S BOTTOM LINE:

Regularly eating dinner together lets you check in on what's really going on with your kids and can get them to eat healthier foods to boot. It may also play a role in keeping your kids away from drugs and alcohol. If schedules make it impossible to sit down together for dinner, don't worry. Carve out another time to connect. It might be weekend lunch or even a once a week or bimonthly "date" with your kids to let them know you care.

27

WILL DOING PUZZLES PREVENT ALZHEIMER'S DISEASE?

There are few conditions as heartbreaking as Alzheimer's disease. I know all too well. My mother-in-law suffered with the disease for almost ten years before her death in 2012. This devastating illness affects not only the patient, but also the families and caregivers. The Alzheimer's Foundation of America defines the condition as "a progressive, degenerative disorder that attacks the brain's nerve cells, or neurons, resulting in loss of memory, thinking and language skills, and behavioral changes." Anyone who's witnessed the devastating decline of people afflicted with the disease knows this clinical description can't begin to capture the sorrow of witnessing a loved one slowly withdraw from the world around them. The disease most often strikes people sixty-five and older, but it can also affect people in their thirties, forties, and fifties. According to the Alzheimer's Association, in 2012, 5.4 million Americans had Alzheimer's disease, affecting roughly one in eight Americans over sixty-five and nearly half of those over eighty-five.

The condition was first identified in 1906 by Dr. Alois Alzheimer, a German physician, whose fifty-one-year-old patient displayed deteriorating memory loss, as well as other dementia symptoms. Upon the patient's death, an autopsy identified in the damaged brain the "plaques and tangles" that now characterize the disease. What's particularly distressing is there is still so little that can be done to treat the disease, apart from easing some of the symptoms.

That brings us to prevention. If you can't do much to treat it, can you do things to prevent it from occurring? Several large studies have looked to see if there are any differences between people who go on to develop Alzheimer's disease and those who don't. One interesting finding was that people who developed Alzheimer's disease were less likely to have done activities like crossword puzzles to stimulate their mind. Could keeping your brain challenged by doing mentally challenging activities ward off memory loss?

Unfortunately, there is only weak scientific evidence that any of these behaviors delays the onset or reduces the severity of the disease. Perhaps the people who developed Alzheimer's disease were less likely to be doing puzzles because they were already having some degree of decline in mental functions. Many people have the disease without realizing it. It can take years to make the diagnosis; there is no simple blood test or X-ray.

This doesn't mean that you won't find all kinds of dietary and behavioral therapies put forward as ways to ward off memory loss. The problem is that the claims far outstrip the evidence. At a 2010 symposium sponsored by the National Institutes of Health (NIH), the "State-of-the-Science Conference on Preventing Alzheimer's Disease and Cognitive Decline," medical, science, and health care experts met to review the existing research. The outcome was discouraging. An NIH press release stated, "Many preventive measures for cognitive decline and for preventing Alzheimer's disease—mental stimulation, exercise, and a variety of dietary supplements—have been studied over the years. However, an independent panel convened this week determined that the value of these strategies for delaying the onset and/or reducing the severity of decline or disease hasn't been demonstrated in rigorous studies."

As the population ages, concerns about Alzheimer's disease grow. There is a greater call for more funding for further studies on prevention and treatment. Until there is more conclusive evidence, what should you do? There's still every reason to make the healthy life choices that are so important as you age. This includes eating a nutritious diet full of fruits and vegetables, staying physically active, not smoking, maintaining a healthy weight, and staying socially connected. These actions can improve your overall health, and if they benefit your brain, all the better.

DR. B'S BOTTOM LINE:

While puzzles aren't proven to prevent Alzheimer's disease, there's no reason not to make every effort to stay mentally alert as you age, for many reasons. Continue to try new things. Take up a musical instrument or other hobby to keep your mind active. While it might not help with this specific disease, it certainly cannot hurt.

28

WILL CONDOMS PREVENT ME FROM GETTING SEXUALLY TRANSMITTED DISEASES (STDs)?

I am a big believer in condom use. Whenever I talk to my patients who are having sex and not in a monogamous relationship, whether they are male or female, they get my condom question. "How often do you have sex without a condom: Rarely, occasionally, or most of the time?" I ask it that way to make it easier for them to tell me the truth. It is pretty unusual for someone to say to me, "Doc, I always use one!" They all know they should be using a condom *every time* they have sex, but unfortunately, it's rare that they do. Condoms not only greatly lower your chances of unwanted pregnancies and the spread of HIV/AIDS; they also can help prevent the spread of many other STDs.

According to the CDC, there are close to nineteen million new STD infections each year. While the highest rate of cases by far is in the twenty-four and younger age group, it's not just adolescents and young adults who are being infected. The rate of disease within older adults has risen. The CDC reports 15 percent of all new HIV/AIDS diagnoses are in adults fifty and over. While adults over forty have the lowest rate of STDs, the rate of disease within that age group has risen significantly—among some diseases even doubled—over the last decade. While this is partially due to more screening, better testing, and population increases in this demographic, it clearly shows that all ages should be conscious of preventing STD transmission.

As much as I try to convince my patients how important it is to their health and the health of their partner, it feels like I'm fighting an uphill battle. Repetition helps: *Condoms only have a chance to work when you wear one.*

Condoms block the transmission of many STDs by acting as a barrier to keep blood, semen, or vaginal fluids, which transmit infections, from passing from one person to another during intercourse. This makes them highly effective against HIV, gonorrhea, chlamydia, and hepatitis B. But not all STDs are spread this way. Some STDs are spread from contact with infected skin. These include genital herpes, syphilis, and human papillomavirus (HPV).

Condoms are the best defense against unwanted diseases, but they can't prevent all STDs 100 percent of the time. So why don't they work all the time? When we talk about condom effectiveness we look at several factors:

- Can the germ get through the condom?
- Is the infection always spread by vaginal or penile secretions?
- How well are the condoms used? Do they break, leak, or slip?

Condoms only reduce the risk for transmission of infections as long as the infected material or area is contained in the condom. Since that isn't always the case, condoms won't always protect you. Then there's oral sex. Some STDs can be spread through mouth contact with the genital area. Any mouth contact directly with vaginal or penile secretions or with infected skin can transmit some STDs.

Lastly, no matter what your age, condoms don't really work if you don't use them properly—every time.

These tips may help:

- Latex (rubber) or polyurethane condoms are more protective than natural (lambskin) condoms, which have larger pores through which some germs can escape.
- Unroll the condom to cover the entire penis, put it on before having sex, and keep it on the entire time. Make sure to remove it carefully so that it doesn't leak or break. The more experienced you are with condoms, the less likely they are to fail.
- Use a new condom every time you have sex. Immediately and carefully remove it after ejaculation.

- Use a water-based lubricant to keep the condom from breaking. Don't use oils or petroleum jelly because they might weaken latex and cause the condom to break.
- Store condoms in a cool, dry place. That means the one that's been in your wallet for years may be no good.

And if you need another reason to practice safe sex, here's an eye-opening one: STDs aren't always easy, or possible, to treat. While we all know that we don't yet have a cure for HIV/AIDS, the difficulty in treating other diseases might be more surprising. Recent headlines raise real fears of resistant strains of gonorrhea, strains almost untreatable with antibiotics. And while herpes often goes dormant, it still is not curable. HPV—which can lead to genital warts and cancer in some—resolves in many, but not all, after a period of years.

Now, I hope this discussion hasn't taken the fun out of having sex—that wasn't the goal. Sex is an important part of a healthy relationship. That being said, it's still necessary to remember that you're never too young, or too old, to take precautions to protect yourself from STDs.

DR. B'S BOTTOM LINE:

If you are sexually active, condoms are your best protection against HIV infection and other STDs, but they aren't foolproof. A properly used condom may not prevent herpes, HPV, or syphilis. If the condom breaks, well then, all bets are off. Even if you are using condoms, if you have had sex with more than one partner, it is extremely important to continue being tested regularly for STDs.

MORE ON SAFE SEX

- Some STDs, such as hepatitis B, hepatitis A, and HPV, can be prevented by vaccination.
- Sometimes an STD has no symptoms at all. For some STDs it's easy to find out your status as well as your partner's. HIV testing can now be done in most doctors' offices in twenty minutes with a simple, painless swab taken from your mouth. Chlamydia and gonorrhea can be tested for in your urine. If you have multiple partners or risk factors for HIV, make sure to get tested at least once a year.

29

CAN USING AN IPOD DAMAGE MY HEARING?

My eighteen-year-old son seems to be permanently attached to his iPod. He even goes to sleep with music in his ears. Does this bother me? You bet it does. As both a father and pediatrician, I am concerned about the disconnect, not just to humanity, but also to everyday dangers like listening for traffic when he walks to school. Most of all, I worry about his future hearing. He is at that age when "future" means tomorrow and concerns even five years away don't register. I remember going to rock concerts when I was his age and leaving the theaters with my ears ringing. That ringing, also known as tinnitus, is a sign of exposure to dangerously high levels of noise. As a teenager, I didn't think anything of it.

These days, it's not just teenagers and young adults who are constantly plugged in and overexposed to noise. Take a good look around the gym, the train, or just on the streets. Everyone has his earbuds in. We're rocking out to music, we're watching YouTube, and we're listening to audiobooks. It's a constant barrage of sound.

While we usually associate hearing loss with the elderly, almost everyone as they age loses some ability to hear, particularly higher-pitched sounds. Some early signs of this type of hearing loss may be an inability to follow a conversation in a noisy restaurant or with the television on. Voices may sound muffled or you may have persistent tinnitus. Unfortunately, this type of hearing loss is being seen more and more commonly in younger people and it is on the rise.

As it is, it's a loud, loud world out there. Every time you walk by an active construction site, cheer at a crowded football stadium, go to a rock concert, or watch a movie in super-surround sound, you risk damage to the sensitive structures in your inner ears, called hair cells. Hair cells convert sound energy into electrical signals that travel along nerves to the brain. Occasional exposure to loud noises damages those hair cells but they bounce back. Repeated overexposure kills them. Once that happens they don't grow back and you are left with noise-induced hearing loss.

So how do you know how loud to play your iPod or other music device? Well, don't use the "no one else can hear it" test. Whether someone can hear your music has as much to do with the type of headphones you use as it does the volume of music. While there are no agreed-upon levels, and what you are exposed to will depend somewhat on your particular device, here are a few tips:

- If you are listening to a personal music device in a loud area, don't turn up your volume to block out background noise, such as other music, construction, subways, or the sound of machines at the gym. You won't be able to recognize that your own volume has reached a dangerous level.
- If you listen in a quiet setting and at a lower volume, you can listen for many hours without causing damage.

DR. B'S BOTTOM LINE:

Using a portable music device can be a wonderful way to enjoy music or other auditory programs. It also provides a constant source of noise that can be damaging to your hearing if you aren't careful. Limit your listening time, dial down the volume, and watch for early signs of hearing loss.

PROTECT YOUR HEARING

- Be aware. If you know what noises can be dangerous, you can work to avoid them or protect yourself.

- Get tested. We frequently get our eyes checked to see if we need glasses, so why not our ears? If you work in a setting where your hearing is at risk, get screened regularly by your doctor. For others, get tested if you have any concerns.
- Be prepared. Bring earplugs to concerts and other venues where the noise might be excessively loud. Even stuffing in cotton balls will help. If you are using loud equipment, such as a lawn mower, wear certified hearing protection.
- Make others aware of the risk. Protect your kids and your friends. Let them know you care by telling them to turn it down, for their own good.

30

WILL USING A HIGHER-NUMBER SUNSCREEN KEEP ME FROM BURNING?

When I stroll down the skin-care aisle in my drugstore to choose a sunscreen I am reminded of a scene in the movie *This Is Spinal Tap*. Nigel Tufnel, the guitarist, is proudly showing off his amplifier, explaining why his is better than anyone else's. While all other amplifiers' volume goes as high as ten, *his* "goes to eleven," making it that much louder than any other. That's sort of how I view sunscreen ratings. They keep going higher and higher looking for their version of eleven, to convince you they are just that bit better than the competition.

We're a nation of sun worshippers and we've paid the price for years of slathering ourselves with coconut-scented oil and baking in the sun. Premature aging of the skin, painful sunburns, and, most worrisome, cancer are the results. According to the NIH, more than two million new cases of skin cancer will be diagnosed this year, more than all other cancers combined. Most are basal cell and squamous cell cancers, the less serious kinds of skin cancers. The big worry is melanoma, cancer arising from the cells that make the pigment in your skin. According to data from the American Cancer Society, in 2012 there were roughly seventy-six thousand new cases of melanoma and more than nine thousand melanoma deaths. And while basal and squamous cell cancers are rarely deadly if treated early, removal can be disfiguring, especially for basal cell cancers that most commonly appear on your face.

Luckily, as we've become more aware of the dangers of excessive sun exposure, we have recognized the importance of using sun protection. There are two types of ultraviolet radiation you should avoid. Ultraviolet B (UVB) rays cause most sunburns and are thought to cause most skin cancers by directly damaging your DNA. Ultraviolet A (UVA) rays, which can also damage cells' DNA, are linked to skin cancer and cause the long-term skin damage associated with aging, such as wrinkles and sunspots. An easy way to remember is A for aging, B for burning.

Sunscreen comes in many strengths, indicated by the sun protection factor (SPF) number. The SPF number is a guide to how much more time, theoretically, you could be in the sun without getting burned by UVB rays. An easy and safe rule of thumb is to gauge how long it normally takes you to burn in the hottest part of the day. Take that amount of time and multiply it by the SPF of your sunscreen. That tells you how much longer you can stay in the sun without burning. Is a higher number always better? Let's see. Without any sunscreen, my wife would normally begin to burn after a half hour. Using a SPF 30 sunscreen allows my wife to stay out thirty times longer. So instead of burning in thirty minutes she would burn in fifteen hours. With my darker skin, I wouldn't burn for an hour, so by using SPF 15 I get the same fifteen hours of protection as she does. One might also think that using a sunscreen with twice as high SPF would block out significantly more UVB rays, but again, there is not as much difference as you would think. SPF 15 sunscreen blocks 93 percent of UVB radiation, SPF 30 blocks nearly 97 percent, and SPF 45 filters out about 98 percent. That suggests enough improvement to warrant going to thirty from fifteen, as most dermatologists recommend, but not necessarily any higher. What about dangerous UVA rays? The SPF number does not address these rays at all. To protect against those dreaded aging UVA rays you need to look for a sunscreen labeled multi-spectrum, broad-spectrum, or UVA/UVB protection. These contain UVA-blocking chemicals such as avobenzone, ecamsule, oxybenzone, zinc oxide, or titanium dioxide.

Thankfully, new sunscreen rules from the FDA have made it a lot easier for all of us to pick a good product by removing some of the misleading advertising that was rampant.

Here are the basics:

- The word *sunblock* is gone! No product blocks all the sun's rays. They now say sunscreen.

- No product can have a number higher than SPF 50. There aren't any data to say that SPF 75 is better than SPF 50, so enough of the numbers game.
- To use the phrase "broad-spectrum" a product has to be at least SPF 15 and provide protection against UVA and UVB rays. While you can't judge how well a product protects against UVA, to use this term, the manufacturer has at least had to convince the FDA.
- No product is waterproof or sweat-proof. Sunscreens are now called water-resistant and must tell you how long they work once you get in the water or start to sweat.
- Any product with an SPF lower than 15 will have a warning label to tell you that it doesn't protect against cancer or early aging.

So now that you picked your number, are you set? Far from it. As with so many other things, you can be your own worst enemy. Several studies show that using a high-numbered sunscreen can create a false sense of security, which leads to a lot of people staying out in the sun much longer than they should. Some experts note that the SPF rating is only the third most important factor when it comes to the usefulness of a particular product. The two most critical ones? Putting on enough sunscreen *and* applying it uniformly and often. The recommended amount is one ounce (one shot glass) for your whole body. Take a look at your bottle and see how long it lasts compared to that suggested use. You'll probably be in for a rude awakening! I sure was.

One more thing. If you have kids, you probably like the spray-on sunscreen that is so easy to apply. The FDA is asking the manufacturers for more data to show that these products really work and whether they are safe if you inhale them.

DR. B'S BOTTOM LINE:

There is no question that sunscreen is an integral part of sun safety. Look for a product that is labeled "broad-spectrum" to get both UVA and UVB coverage. Just remember, none offers 100 percent protection. Even an SPF 50 sunscreen is of little use if it is not used properly. And lastly, a little bit of sun each day is good for you. It's how our bodies make vitamin D.

STANDING UP TO THE SUN

Think of sunscreen as just one component in your battle against sunburn, sun damage, and skin cancer. Before that thin film of protection becomes all that stands between you and the sun, make sure you take all other necessary precautions:

- Try to limit your time in the sun when the sun is at its zenith, generally from 10 a.m. to 4 p.m.
- Generously apply sunscreen fifteen to thirty minutes before going outdoors to allow it time to penetrate.
- Protect your skin even on cool or overcast days. Although you won't feel the heat, the sun's rays are still doing as much damage as on a sunny day.
- Australia had a successful, and easy to remember, program called "slip, slop, and slap." Slip on a shirt, slop on sunscreen, slap on a wide-brimmed hat. While you're at it, add some sunglasses with UV protection and an umbrella at the beach.
- Take special care when using skin-care products with retinol or certain antibiotics. They can make your skin more sensitive to sunlight.
- Have regular mole and skin checks with your dermatologist. If you have a history of skin cancer in your family, you are at higher risk as well.

31

CAN I CATCH A COLD FROM BEING IN A CHILLING RAIN?

We've all been there. The runny nose that just won't stop. The stuffy head, pounding, pounding, pounding. Sinuses that feel like they are about to explode. Red and itchy eyes. A scratchy and raw throat crying out for relief. Is there any misery worse than that oh so "common" cold?

When it comes to prevention, I bet you, like I, have heard them all. They all start with *don't*—but everyone has her favorite: Don't get caught in the rain, don't go to bed with wet hair, don't sit near a draft, don't go out in the cold without a coat. You get the idea . . .

These old wives' tales have traveled down through the generations. From the time we were toddlers, we've been told by our grandmothers, mothers, and fathers to heed those warnings. Now a parent, even I have to restrain myself from scolding my son as he heads to school wearing a T-shirt on a thirty-degree day. It's become an automatic response, although it's been shown in study after study to be false. Colds aren't caused by cold temperatures, and there is little to suggest your immune system is compromised when you get your hair wet or catch a chill.

Before we talk about why this idea persists, let's just review the basics. Getting any infection involves the interaction of three factors: The germ, the person, and the environment. Colds are caused by viruses that we pass between each other. That's the germ part of it. Ever wonder why some people never catch a cold and some catch them all? Some people have stronger immune systems, wash their hands more often, or have less exposure than others. That's the person part. Then there is the environment. Many environmental factors determine how easy it is for a cold virus to pass from person to person. The closer we are to each other, the more easily viruses spread.

Instead of blaming the cold or rainy weather, blame those germs your colleagues or children so kindly shared. Sometimes they're passed to you by coughs or sneezes. More often they are spread by hand-to-hand contact when a sick person touches his nose, eyes, or other infected area (or sneezes into her hands), and then touches you or something you are about to touch.

Now that we are on the same page about the factors involved in cold virus transmission, let's return to the big question: Whether being chilled and wet leads to catching a cold. Theories about the relationship of cold and frigid weather go as far back as the nineteenth century. But studies have shown no relationship between *being* cold and *getting* a cold. Some researchers went so far as to smear cold viruses into the noses of people and then divide them into two groups. One group was exposed to chilling cold temperatures while the others were kept warm and toasty. There was no difference in the rate of individuals contracting a cold between the two groups.

So why does this notion persist? It is fueled in large part by circumstantial evidence. In the United States and many other parts of the world, the majority of colds occur during the cooler fall and winter months, when people are in more confined spaces, making it easier for germs to spread. As anyone with children knows, kids in packed schoolrooms pass germs back and forth constantly. The winter holidays are busy times, leaving you stressed, sleep-deprived, and run-down. We congregate in malls and planes to shop and travel. Additionally, cold viruses transmit better when there is lower humidity. Less humidity also makes the inside lining of your nose drier and more vulnerable to infection.

Ultimately, whether we make our loved ones bundle up and keep dry as a health precaution or simply because we want them to stay warm and snug, we're doing them no harm (except for, as my kids would say, "being so annoying"). This is one of those times when adhering to personal beliefs that have no medical credence does no damage to your well-being, so I am inclined to let it slide. At some level it is really us just saying, I love you and want to keep you well.

DR. B'S BOTTOM LINE:

If you want to avoid catching the common cold, focus on practicing good hand hygiene, keeping away from people who are sick, and doing what it takes to preserve a healthy immune system, rather than bundling up or cranking up the thermostat. You'll be much better off.

A COLD SURVIVAL GUIDE

When you have a cold, help yourself feel better and prevent others from catching it by following this advice.

- Don't ask for an antibiotic! Colds are caused by viruses; antibiotics work against bacteria. Taking antibiotics when you have a cold can set you up for a resistant bacterial infection and won't make your cold go away faster.
- Model good behavior. Stop shaking hands when you're sick. If you are really sick, don't go to work. Believe me, no one wants you to "tough it out," especially if you could cause them to catch your bug.
- Drink lots of liquids. As your body loses moisture through secretions, you might become dehydrated. I like to drink warm liquids when I am congested or have a sore throat. Chicken soup and tea with honey, lemon and crushed fresh ginger are my favorites. Others prefer to ease the pain of a sore throat with Popsicles and cold drinks. Do what works for you.
- Gargling with salt water and sucking on lozenges can also ease the discomfort of a raw throat.
- A steamy shower can open up your nasal passages and help you breathe, especially in the morning when you wake up congested.

- Take it easy. Get plenty of sleep and give your body a break so that it can heal itself. It's good to give your eyes, throat, and brain a rest.
- Use moisturizer to soothe the skin around your nose when it becomes raw.
- Try an over-the-counter fever medication if you are uncomfortable with the fever (but remember that low-grade fever isn't dangerous and can help your immune system fight the virus).

32

IS RELIGION GOOD FOR MY HEALTH?

Faith and medicine frequently intersect. My patients and I often talk about spirituality when we discuss medical issues. For many people, life-and-death decisions are grounded in a belief that a higher being will guide the outcome as much, or more than, the physicians and treatments involved. In addition, a support system based on shared faith can be extremely helpful in the healing process. Ministries frequently offer assistance programs and have relationships with social workers to counsel and provide services for those in need.

Not long ago, while reading the newspaper, I began thinking about the relationship of health and religion in an entirely new way, one that involves using religious tenets to promote a healthful lifestyle every day, not just in times of crisis. I saw an obituary for Lester Breslow, a true pioneer in public health. It was fitting that a man who dedicated his life to understanding what drives longevity lived to the ripe old age of ninety-seven. There are many important lessons to be learned from his extensive body of research. Breslow, a public health leader for more than seventy years, was instrumental in first connecting smoking to lung diseases, particularly cancer. But that's not all. He demonstrated an association between longevity and health quality through a set of seven behaviors (known as the Alameda 7, for the California county in which they were identified): Not smoking; sleeping seven to eight hours per night; eating regular meals; maintaining a moderate weight; eating breakfast; drinking in moderation; and exercising at least moderately.

What really caught my eye was that Dr. Breslow was still at work well into his nineties. In 2010, Breslow, then ninety-five, was a coauthor of a twenty-five-year study of a group of California Mormons. This study, written with Professor James E. Enstrom of the University of California, Los Angeles, showed that the life expectancy of Mormon men was almost ten years longer than that of the general population of white American males. Female Mormons lived between five and six years longer than their general population counterparts. The longevity effect was most pronounced for those who never smoked, who went to church weekly, had at least twelve years of education, and were married. Additional benefits were seen in those who were not overweight, got plenty of sleep, and exercised. The authors attributed the added years to the Mormons' healthy doctrines: Eating a well-balanced diet and eschewing tobacco, alcohol, coffee, tea, and illegal drugs. They found similar benefits among Americans of any religion who practiced the same healthy behaviors.

There has long been a correlation between being a churchgoer and longevity, but it has been difficult to tease out the basis of that relationship. The link to better health was partially attributed to self-selection. Religious people were the type of people who would practice behaviors favorable to more healthful living and thus live longer. Studies found that churchgoers were less likely to engage in high-risk health behaviors such as smoking and excessive drinking. After all, getting up bright and early for church Sunday mornings does hamper Saturday night bingeing. Being able to travel to church might also be a marker for mobility and healthfulness, rather than its cause.

There are also many beneficial spiritual aspects to consider. The meditative nature of religious services can lower stress levels. Many services preach love, forgiveness, hope, and optimism, which foster a positive outlook on life that can translate into good emotional health. Many sermons address the importance of giving thanks, and we know that gratitude can be very important for mental health. In addition to religious leaders providing counseling, some religions incorporate confession, which can help unburden congregants from emotional distress. These are all things that might be good for your health.

Now, I'm not a religious person and I've yet to see any convincing studies that compare the belief systems of various religions and their impact on health. However, I know from experience that for some people the belief in a higher power is incredibly important in helping them cope with a serious illness. It is what gets them through tough times. For others, it is the sense of community, the group aspect of organized religion that has a big impact on their health. Alternatively, I see atheists who get great support through other means, including their understanding of the natural workings of the world. And clearly you don't need to be religious to practice the healthful principles laid out by many of the world's religions. Those should apply to everyone.

DR. B'S BOTTOM LINE:

Practicing the health tenets espoused by many religions is associated with a longer life. And you know what? You don't need to be religious or believe in God to follow them!

KEEPING THE FAITH

Even if you aren't religious, it's worth embracing some philosophies espoused by many faith-based organizations that are good for your health and the health of others:

- Find a loving relationship and stick with it.
- Support those around you in their times of need.
- Give thanks for what you have. There are many benefits of being grateful. It has been shown to strengthen social bonds and makes people more likely to want to help us again. There is also promising evidence linking practicing gratitude to better sleep, fewer symptoms of illness, and less stress.
- Stay in school. Education is good for your health.
- Treat your body like a temple. Eat right, get regular exercise, get a good night's sleep, don't smoke, and if you drink, do so in moderation.

33

IS ANTIBACTERIAL SOAP BETTER THAN PLAIN SOAP?

Confession time. I am a bit obsessed with clean hands. People who know me know that if you ask me for hand sanitizer, nine times out of ten I'll have some in my pocket. If I don't, I'll know where you can get some quickly. If you see me around, try me.

Why do I care so much about handwashing? Easy. The simplest way to pick up an unwanted infection is by touching someone's hands that are contaminated with germs. It's not the only way. Someone with a virus can sneeze or cough in your face (a common occurrence for me as a pediatrician); you can eat contaminated food; you can be bitten by a mosquito carrying West Nile virus; and you can have unprotected sex with someone who has a sexually transmitted disease. Believe me, there are many ways to pick up diseases, but by far, hands are the way you are going to pick up the majority of your infections.

When I was acting director of the CDC in 2009, the swine flu pandemic was spreading across the country and around the world. We had a terrific communications team that spread messages detailing what people could do to protect themselves. A key message: Wash your hands. One of the most rewarding things we saw during that health crisis was that the recommendation took hold. Around the country people were taking this to heart, trying to prevent the infection from spreading.

Now, if handwashing is good, shouldn't handwashing with antibacterial soaps be better? Actually, no. But it's easy to see why you would think otherwise. Over the past few decades, manufacturers have been marketing antibacterial soap and other antibacterial products as a better way to wash and protect yourself. They've tried to convince consumers that soap is not enough. You need something stronger, special "bacteria-fighting" soap, to truly kill germs. You can see the power of that marketing on store shelves. Antibacterial products have crowded out traditional soaps. Trying to find a bottle of plain liquid soap is nearly impossible.

Unlike regular soap, antibacterial soaps contain chemicals, frequently triclosan, triclocarban, and benzalkonium chloride. Unless you have an immune deficiency, there is no reason to use a soap containing an antibacterial chemical. Numerous studies have shown this. One of my favorites was done by my friend Dr. Steve Luby, in Pakistan. His research group wanted to see whether handwashing reduced the stomach flu in children and whether doing so with antibacterial soap was even better. They randomly assigned people in neighborhoods to wash their hands with soap, wash them with antibacterial soap, or continue whatever their current practice was. They found that both handwashing and handwashing with antibacterial soap reduced stomach flu by more than 50 percent, but surprisingly, antibacterial soap was absolutely no better than plain old soap. What really blew me away was this: Many of these villages didn't even have clean water. Handwashing even works when the water isn't clean. Just the friction of the soap and water can reduce germs.

I really worry about antibacterial agents in soaps. In the laboratory, triclosan can promote antibiotic resistance. While this hasn't been demonstrated in people using soaps with triclosan, why expose yourself to chemicals without getting any added benefit?

What about those times when you don't have access to running water and soap? Go with an alcohol-based hand sanitizer with at least 60 percent alcohol. But if you see dirt on your hands, don't think the sanitizer is going to get the job done.

DR. B'S BOTTOM LINE:

Handwashing is one of those little things you can do every day that makes a big difference to your health. You'll see this advice mentioned in this book over and over again. The best way to protect yourself from colds, flu, and other illnesses is to wash your hands with good old-fashioned soap. It doesn't take long but you need to do it right.

ARE YOUR HANDS REALLY CLEAN?

To make sure that you're washing your hands adequately:

- Rub your hands together vigorously to make a lather and scrub all surfaces. Continue for twenty seconds. That's longer than you think. It takes that long for the soap and scrubbing action to dislodge and remove stubborn germs. Need a mental timer? Imagine singing "Happy Birthday" all the way through—twice.
- When in a public restroom, if possible use your paper towel to turn off the faucet and open the door. That way, your clean hands will stay that way a little bit longer.

34

HOW DO I PROTECT MYSELF FROM GERMS?

Face it: We live in a pretty germy world. Although they are invisible to us, we are surrounded and outnumbered by bacteria, viruses, and parasites that can make us sick. But for most people, the one place where hygiene concerns really rule is in the bathroom. Who hasn't heard the murmurs from moms to kids warning, "Don't touch anything," when they use a public restroom? This is pretty good advice. However, there are more germs on the items you touch without a second thought at home and at the office than in most bathrooms. A British consumer advocacy group commissioned a microbiologist to compare swabs from thirty-three keyboards, a toilet seat, and a toilet door handle at their office. He found one of the keyboards tested had levels of germs five times higher than that found on the toilet seat.

Before you go out and buy up all the hydrogen peroxide you can find to try to sterilize your world, know that not all germs are created equal. Many bacteria play critical roles in maintaining your health. Some are important for digestion. Ever wonder why many antibiotics give you diarrhea? It's because they kill off *helpful* bacteria that are important in digestion. Other bacteria in our intestines provide our bodies with vitamin K, essential for normal clotting of our blood. And when it comes to bacteria that cause disease, some don't live very long on surfaces. Other bacteria live for a long time but are harmless. These germs can be cultured off of many common surfaces, but they are unlikely to make you sick.

So while many of the items in your home or office might have more germs, we are right to focus on the bathroom because many dangerous infections are spread through the fecal-oral route. Germs are shed into your bowel movements, and when you don't use good hygiene, they also get onto your hands. From there they can pass to everything you touch. If you touch unclean surfaces in the bathroom and then your mouth, you may be ingesting dangerous germs. So while the actual *numbers* of germs may be lower, the ones you find in the bathroom should be taken seriously. On the other hand, bathrooms also get regularly cleaned with disinfectant. Can you remember the last time you sanitized your TV remote or telephone?

If you want to stay healthy, rather than focusing so much on surfaces that may contain germs, think more about how germs get into your body and aim to reduce it. To do that, once again, you will clearly want to look at your hands. They are the germs' best friends. Why? The most common way to spread and contract viruses is to touch contaminated hands or surfaces and then touch your face. Your mouth, nose, and eyes are the doors through which these nasty germs enter.

Not long after I got to ABC News we decided to do a little experiment to look at how easily germs spread. We secretly filmed a staff meeting full of producers during flu season. We counted the number of times people touched their noses and mouths. When the staff watched the replay even they were shocked. One producer touched his nose, mouth, or eyes 44 times in just 25 minutes. They all touched their faces at least once. Guess what they all did when they left the meeting—they went about their day, drinking from the water fountain, using the communal microwave and fridge, answering phones, and typing away on keyboards. Where do you think all the germs on their hands went? On the things we touch all the time, never suspecting that they might harbor disease.

Here's the best way to protect yourself. After you use the bathroom, before you eat, and when you get up in the morning, wash your hands. Keeping your hands clean reduces the spread of infection and illness and helps prevent you from getting sick. Again, when soap and water aren't available, those alcohol-based hand sanitizers with at least 60 percent alcohol are a good option. I keep a dispenser on my desk. You should, too.

DR. B'S BOTTOM LINE:

Germs are everywhere, but not all germs are the same. Instead of focusing on sterilizing your world, take some simple steps to keep high-risk areas clean. Wash your hands often—it's your best protection against germs.

YOU CAN'T STERILIZE YOUR WORLD, BUT YOU CAN MAKE IT A BIT SAFER

Sterilizing your world doesn't make sense, but keeping these areas clean does. A wipe-down with a disinfectant spray or dilute bleach solution—a stronger bleach concentration is recommended for bathrooms than for kitchens—will take care of most of the germs that can cause disease.

- Kitchen: In particular the food preparation areas.
- Pet food area: Some pet foods can harbor salmonella. Wash your hands well after handling dry pet food.
- Bathroom surfaces
- Diaper changing area

35

IS A DRINK OR TWO A DAY GOOD FOR ME?

When it comes to alcohol consumption, the fine line between indulgence and overindulgence can be a difficult and contentious one to establish. One person's idea of being a social drinker is another's definition of a fall-down drunk. Because of the subjective nature, it can be delicate to talk about drinking as being potentially advantageous to your health.

I'm a drink-a-day kind of guy. I admit it—when I get home from work I unwind with a cocktail, beer, or glass of wine. I like the flavor, I like the breath of relaxation it brings as I transition from my workday to home, and I like that I'm most likely doing something that is good for my health. Going back over more than forty years, there are dozens of studies that suggest a connection between moderate alcohol consumption and various measures of good health—particularly when it comes to preventing heart disease, stroke, and diabetes. Not only do moderate drinkers have lower risks of heart disease, but when they do have a heart attack, they are less likely to die from it than heavy drinkers or those who don't drink at all.

Here may be the reason why. Moderate amounts of alcohol raise your good cholesterol and may prevent platelets, the component in your blood that helps to form clots, from clumping together. Both of these actions tend to reduce plaque formation in your arteries, which lowers your risk of heart attack and stroke.

However, many of the findings on the benefits of alcohol come from weak studies and offer soft proof at best. Here's why: Some research suggests that this seeming connection between alcohol consumption and heart benefits has less to do with the health effects of alcohol and more to do with the characteristics of the people who drink it on occasion. I call this the "chicken and egg" quandary, and it is typical of medical research. Are people who drink moderately also more likely to have other qualities that could influence their health? Might judicious drinkers be more likely to stop eating when they are full or say no to dessert? For alcohol benefit studies, these questions are critical.

This is really important but difficult to sort out. The gold standard in medical research is something called a double-blinded randomized controlled trial. In this type of study, you take a group of people and randomly assign them to either take the drug of interest or a placebo, something that looks like the drug but doesn't contain any active substance. Neither the researchers nor the participants know who is assigned to which group, until the end of the study. At that point you look for differences in the health outcomes. The random assignment is also important because other behaviors that may be linked to developing disease—such as being overweight, smoking, having high blood pressure—get evenly assigned as well.

In a perfect world, if I wanted to study whether moderate alcohol consumption reduced the risk of heart disease, I would take a large group of people (probably thousands) and randomly assign them to drink moderately or not. Then, after about ten years, I would look at health outcomes. Clearly it would be unethical to do this study since there are so many downsides to drinking alcohol, but it would definitively answer the study question.

Since we can't do these studies we are left with doing what are called observational studies. We compare people who have heart attacks or heart disease with those who don't and look to see if there are any differences in how much alcohol they normally drink. It is a less definitive type of study since you then need to take into account, through statistical manipulation, differences in other known risk factors for heart disease.

My read of the evidence is this: I do think that there is a health benefit from moderate consumption of alcohol, but not enough to recommend that someone who doesn't drink start. The American Heart Association, which uniformly stands behind heart-healthy lifestyle adjustments, agrees; don't start to drink just to protect yourself from heart problems. As we all know, drinking has its own inherent risks. According to the CDC there are seventy-nine thousand deaths and more than one and a half million hospitalizations in the United States each year linked to alcohol overuse.

Health consequences include motor vehicle accidents, liver disease, domestic violence, birth defects, high blood pressure, and alcohol abuse and addiction. There are also some studies that point to an increased risk of breast cancer from moderate alcohol consumption. While the increase is slight, if you are at high risk for breast cancer, you might want to factor this into your decision.

If you are a drinker already, how much is the right amount? As I said, I'm a drink-a-day fellow—that's "a" as in one or if I'm out for dinner, two. The U.S. Department of Agriculture (USDA) defines moderate drinking as one drink per day for women and up to two drinks per day for men. What is one drink? Probably less than you think. For wine, five ounces, less than an average juice glass. (Use a measuring cup and compare it to where you normally fill your wineglass. You could be surprised.) Beer is a typical twelve-ounce bottle. Hard liquor, typically eighty-proof distilled spirits such as vodka, is defined as 1½ ounces—again, not your typical bartender pour. For the heart-healthy benefits described, I am talking about *per day* drinking. You can't store up your one glass a day to equal seven drinks on Saturday night.

Like many medical decisions, there is no clear-cut answer that applies to everyone. You need to weigh your own risks and benefits, taking into account family history of heart disease, alcohol abuse, and breast cancer. I feel that for me, having a drink a day, perhaps even a couple on some days, is fairly safe—and it may even have health benefits, particularly when it comes to cardiovascular health.

DR. B'S BOTTOM LINE:

Take the advice of the American Heart Association: If you drink moderately already, keep it to a drink or two a day. If you don't drink, don't start doing so for supposed health reasons.

36

DO ADULTS NEED SHOTS?

Katie and Craig Van Tornhout tried desperately to have a baby. I reported on their heart-wrenching story for *Good Morning America* several years ago. After four miscarriages, Katie finally had success. The pregnancy went smoothly; her obstetrician made sure she had her flu shot; and on Christmas day, Callie Grace was born. They called her their miracle baby. A couple of weeks later, Callie Grace developed a cough. Her pediatrician checked her out and didn't think it was anything serious. The cough didn't get better and after a few days her worried parents took her back to the doctor's office. While there, Callie Grace stopped breathing. Although they were able to revive her, it wasn't for long. At just thirty-eight days old, Callie Grace died. The cause was whooping cough, also known as pertussis, a contagious bacterial infection that can be prevented by vaccination.

Katie had no idea that the whooping cough vaccine was recommended for women during pregnancy who had not already received it as an adult. The protective antibodies from receiving the vaccine pass through the placenta and protect babies during the first four months of life. They will never know how Callie Grace came in contact with pertussis, but they do know that Katie never had the chance to provide her with protection. You get vaccinated for two reasons: To protect yourself from infections and to protect those around you who can't protect themselves. Many people think of vaccinations as something just for kids, something that you don't need to worry about except for the annual flu shot. Unfortunately, those adults are wrong and are putting themselves and others at risk.

By the time you are eighteen years old, you will have hopefully received your recommended battery of childhood vaccines and booster shots that protects against sixteen different diseases. The number of actual shots varies from patient to patient depending on whether you get combination vaccines. A comprehensive schedule of all recommended childhood vaccinations can be found on this Web page of the U.S. Centers for Disease Control and Prevention: www.cdc.gov/vaccines/schedules/downloads/child /0-18yrs-11x17-fold-pr.pdf.

For children, vaccine recommendations are pretty straightforward. Almost all children get the same vaccines and need to have proof of vaccination to enter school. For adults, it's a bit different. What vaccines you need depends somewhat on your age, underlying health condition, occupation, and potential exposures. There are fourteen vaccines that are recommended for adults, and while few adults need them all, every adult needs at least one.

Here they are:

- **Influenza (flu):** Anyone over age six months should get an annual flu vaccination. While the quality of protection from the vaccine varies year to year, presently this is the best approach to reducing your chance of getting the flu.
- **Tetanus, diphtheria, and pertussis (whooping cough):** Most adults know that they need to get a tetanus shot every ten years (and not just when they step on a nail). However, most don't know that one of the boosters should also contain protection against pertussis. We are seeing a rise in the number of cases of whooping cough each year, perhaps due to falling immunity among adults and teenagers. All tetanus vaccines also contain protection against diphtheria.
- **Varicella (chicken pox):** All adults without evidence of immunity (documentation of two shots, born before 1980, history of having had chicken pox, or blood test showing antibodies) should get vaccinated. Normal series is two shots, spaced four to eight weeks apart.
- **Human papillomavirus (HPV):** A vaccine that prevents cancer! Fantastic! This virus causes cervical cancer, genital cancer, anal cancer, oral cancer, and genital warts. The vaccine protects against the strains of HPV most responsible for cancer and is recommended for all men and women through age twenty-six. The series is three shots given over six months.

- **Zoster (shingles):** This one-time vaccine is recommended for all adults sixty years and older.
- **Pneumococcal vaccine (pneumonia):** This vaccine offers some protection against certain types of pneumonia and bloodstream infections. It is routinely given to adults sixty-five and older and to younger adults with certain medical conditions, including lung disease, heart disease, diabetes, and immune disorders.
- **Meningococcal vaccine (meningitis):** This vaccine is given to teenagers and young adults up to twenty-one. It is also recommended for people traveling to parts of the world where epidemic meningitis is common.
- **Hepatitis A:** Young children get this routinely but if you are an adult, odds are you didn't get it. If you are in a group at increased risk for hepatitis A, including men who have sex with men, food handlers, and people traveling to underdeveloped countries, go ahead and get vaccinated. This is a two-vaccine series.
- **Hepatitis B:** This is a devastating disease that can cause liver failure, cirrhosis, liver cancer, and death. Another cancer vaccine! All children receive this vaccine; most start shortly after birth. However, this hasn't always been the case. If you are an adult there is a good chance you were never vaccinated. Make sure you are protected.
- **Measles, mumps, rubella (MMR):** Children in the United States are routinely given two doses of this vaccine. However, many adults have received only one shot. Get a second dose if you are in college or university, work in a health care facility, or will be doing any international travel. These diseases are much more prevalent in some other parts of the world and travelers returning home continue to trigger outbreaks in the United States.

The next time you see your doctor, ask about immunizations. Explore the CDC website before you go. Keep a running record of what you've had and when, but if you aren't sure what you've had, get it again. No harm there.

DR. B'S BOTTOM LINE:

Adults need vaccinations, too. With new vaccines being recommended all the time and more vaccines needed as we age, make sure to bring the list in this section to review with your doctor. Not being up to date on your vaccines can be a big problem, both for you and for those around you.

4

MEDICINE CABINET: FRIEND OR FOE?

Your Questions on Vitamins, Supplements, and Medications

There's no doubt about it: We're pill-popping people. There are pills for when we're sick, pills for when we're healthy, and pills for when we're just not sure. Our medicine cabinets have become "junk drawers," stuffed full of half-filled bottles just in case we need them down the road.

Why are we so dependent on pills for everything? It's all about the easy fix. No time to eat nutritiously? No problem, just take a multivitamin. Feeling the sniffles? Run for the vitamin C. But will these help? The vitamin and supplement industry has made every effort to convince you they will. I worry that a blind belief in these treatments might keep you from doing the things that can truly help your health. But if these supplements aren't improving your health, wouldn't your money be better spent on something that has been proven to do so, like a gym membership or more healthful food? I think so.

While advancements in drug development have saved countless lives, drugs can be incredibly dangerous if used by the wrong people or in the wrong way. And far too often they are. So many questions surround even over-the-counter medications. Are all painkillers created equal? Are generics as good as name brands? If there's a chance aspirin can stave off serious conditions such as cancer, heart disease, and stroke, shouldn't we all just take it? In this chapter, you'll learn what you need to do to make the best choices for you. You'll learn the critical questions you need to ask before you pop any pill.

The old days of "take two and call me in the morning" are over—or should be. All medications have risks and it's important that you be aware of them. Even over-the-counter painkillers, if overused, can cause serious injury or death. The truth is that when it comes to medicines, one size does not fit all.

37

SHOULD I TAKE A DAILY MULTIVITAMIN?

There is perhaps no more ubiquitous bottle in the American home than the one that holds the multivitamins. According to a 2011 report by the CDC, about 40 percent of American adults take one daily. My friend is one of them. He lives on a diet of frozen dinners and candy. No fresh vegetables, no fruits. When I tell him I'm concerned about his health, he says not to worry; he takes a multivitamin every day. To him it's a kind of health insurance. When I questioned that approach, he got pretty darn defensive. For believers, taking multivitamins is a sensitive subject. They feel they are doing something critically important for their health. When I tell friends I have never taken a multivitamin, they're shocked. Surely as a doctor, I should be more responsible about my health, they say. I reply that I get my vitamins through eating a balanced diet, but it's clear they just don't believe me.

Why are Americans spending billions of dollars on multivitamins every year? Probably several reasons. Since you were little you've been told to take your vitamins and in fact, vitamins *are* essential for life. Vitamin C deficiency causes scurvy, niacin deficiency causes pellagra, vitamin A deficiency can lead to blindness, and vitamin D deficiency causes rickets. No one wants to be vitamin-deficient. The big questions are whether having extra vitamins is a good thing and whether getting vitamins through pills is equivalent to getting them from your food. Also, are multivitamins really as important to your health as advertisements would lead you to believe? The current science suggests that the answer to this question is probably not.

Most of the evidence suggests that taking a multivitamin won't help you live any longer than not taking one. Many studies have tried to sort this out and most are observational studies or association studies, the same type of studies I talked about in the question about whether having a drink a day is good for you. These studies look at a group of people over time to see whether those who took vitamins had better or worse health outcomes. Their results vary widely; some show slight benefits, but others show increased risks of death.

An expert panel convened in 2006 to give advice to the NIH on the research supporting vitamins for the prevention of chronic disease. They concluded that the present evidence was "insufficient to recommend either for or against the use" of multivitamins. The U.S. Preventive Services Task Force reached the same conclusion. That's a bit surprising given the enthusiasm so many people have for them and the advertising that suggests they are absolutely essential for maintaining health. If vitamins are so vital, why is it so hard to show a benefit to your health?

Although I don't support general use of multivitamins and supplements, I am a big fan of eating a diet rich in vitamins and other nutrients. I worry that divorcing these vitamins from the foods from which they naturally come implies that they are somehow just as, if not more, effective in pill form. Additionally, although some vitamins taken in excess are simply eliminated in the urine, many vitamins taken in high doses have been shown to be harmful. The good news is that your body stores vitamins to be used at times when they aren't available in your diet. As long as you are eating a balanced diet most of the time, you should get enough.

It is pretty easy to find someone who will tell you that you need to take more vitamins. For a segment on *Good Morning America*, I went on two popular vitamin websites to see what they would try to sell me. To set the stage, I repeat, I eat a very healthful diet. As a family we eat a wide variety of foods and plenty of fruits and vegetables every day. I have no chronic medical conditions and thankfully, no family history of early heart disease. Both sites felt I needed to do a lot more. One site recommended I take a daily antioxidant, a daily multivitamin, B-50, vitamin C, omega-3 fatty acids, and a special supplement! The cost: $600 per year. Another website had similar recommendations: Vitamin C, calcium, fish oil with vitamin E, magnesium, vitamin D, super B, milk thistle, and a multivitamin! Their price: $624 per year. Think about that. Even with my concerted effort to eat a balanced diet, vitamin companies still suggest that I need to spend more than $600 in supplements. Just imagine what the recommendation would be for someone a little less conscientious. It could easily go into the four figures. You could be doing so many other things with that money!

I don't want to go on a rant here, but there is more pseudoscience attached to the vitamin and supplement industry than just about anywhere in health care. It is an industry that needs more effective governmental oversight to protect the public.

DR. B'S BOTTOM LINE:

We spend billions of dollars on multivitamins every year. Take the money you are spending on them and put it toward eating more servings of healthy fruits and vegetables. It's not only a more straightforward approach to the vitamins and minerals you need, but it can be a tastier one, too.

WHO NEEDS A MULTIVITAMIN?

There are some exceptions to the rule when it comes to multivitamins and health benefits.

- Women who are pregnant or planning to get pregnant should take a pregnancy multivitamin.
- Some people with chronic medical conditions that impair absorption of specific foods will need specific vitamin supplements.
- People on diets deficient in certain nutrients (vegans, for example) may need a particular vitamin rather than a multivitamin.

38

WILL TAKING VITAMIN C PREVENT ME FROM GETTING A COLD?

I hate getting a cold. Who doesn't? As a pediatrician, I have had more than most adults. It never fails: I'll be looking into the back of a sick child's throat and he'll take that moment to hit me with a major sneeze or cough. That's it! A few days later I feel the early signs and I know I'll be a bit miserable for the next week or so. Just like you, I sure wish there was something I could do when I know I've been exposed, or during the peak season, to prevent colds from happening. Unfortunately, there is no magic bullet.

There's enough mythology around cold prevention and treatment to fill an entire book. One of the most popular theories—that excess vitamin C wards off colds—goes back more than forty years, to Linus Pauling, a two-time Nobel Prize–winning biologist, who began promoting supplemental vitamin C for the prevention of colds. Since then, scores of studies have concluded that regular use of vitamin C does not reduce the frequency of colds in the general population.

Some people like the "just in case" approach to health care. That's where you say, "I'll take it just in case." I am not a fan of that tactic, for many reasons. First, relying on treatments that haven't been proven to work can lead to confusion as to what is based on science and what is based on faith. Better to make decisions based on evidence. While there are some studies that show that adults who take at least 200 mg of vitamin C every day have slightly shorter colds (less than twelve hours shorter), that's not enough of a lure for me to take it throughout cold season. For those of you who are attracted to those ever so slightly shorter colds, and are willing to take pills every day "just in case," there is some good news. Vitamin C is relatively safe at low doses. If you keep your intake in the lower range, I don't think you are doing any harm—even if studies suggest you aren't doing much good. What your body doesn't use will be excreted in your urine.

What about taking vitamin C after you get a cold, to diminish its length or intensity? I can't tell you how many people at work rush for their emergency mega-doses of vitamin C when they get a cold. Sorry, but there is only bad news in that department. Taking vitamin C after the cold starts doesn't work.

DR. B'S BOTTOM LINE:

As frustrating as it is, there really is no pill to prevent the common cold. Taking vitamin C religiously won't prevent the common cold, though it might shorten it just a little bit. Taking vitamin C after a cold has started doesn't do a thing. Best to focus on trying to prevent a cold in the first place.

KEEPING COLDS AT BAY

To keep healthy during cold season, try the following tried-and-true ways to prevent colds:

- Wash your hands, wash your hands, wash your hands. The best way to prevent illnesses is to wash your hands with soap and warm water frequently. If you are not near a sink, use sanitizing gel or alcohol-based hand wipes.
- Get at least seven or eight hours of sleep. The more rested you are the better your body can fight infection.
- Eat right. Strengthen your immune system by eating a balanced diet.
- Stay active. Keep your immune system revved by keeping fit. If you're at the gym, make sure to wipe down the machines with a sanitizing wipe before and after using them.
- Keep your distance. If you see someone sneezing and coughing—stay clear. Conversely, if you aren't feeling well, stay away from others.

- Teach your family where to sneeze. To prevent the spread of germs, sneeze and cough into the crook of your elbow, or a tissue, not into your hands. Throw the tissue away after each use.
- Encourage healthy workplace policies. It is hard to do the right thing if you don't have sick days for yourself and to care for family members. Encourage family leave policies.

39

SHOULD I TAKE A DAILY ASPIRIN TO PREVENT A HEART ATTACK, STROKE, OR CANCER?

It used to be, "An apple a day keeps the doctor away." Now it seems like aspirin has pushed the beloved ruby icon of health aside.

During my training, the chairman of the pediatric department gave me a great piece of advice. He said, "You never want to be the first one to adopt a new therapy . . . but you also don't want to be the last." You don't want to be first, because when new drugs come on the market or new treatments are implemented, there is less understanding of what their serious side effects and long-term consequences might be. New treatments all look fantastic until they are tried on millions of people. All too often, after further evaluation, products that once seemed promising are found not to be helpful, and sometimes are actually harmful. On the flip side, you don't want to be last, because in doing so you may deny your patients innovative treatments that have proven their worth. Bridging this dichotomy of informed decision making drives much of my approach to medicine. The goal is to be skeptical of new treatments but open to being convinced.

We've all heard the advice somewhere: Take a baby aspirin every day to lessen the risk of heart attack or stroke. It's tantalizingly easy to follow. After all, aspirin is available over-the-counter, is universally known, and has been used by nearly everyone at one time or another. Additionally, we hear all the time about how more Americans die from heart disease than from any other illness. Stroke is not that far behind.

The temptation to take a daily baby aspirin, without a doctor's advice, might not seem like such a bad idea. After all, everyone's doing it—and how bad can a baby aspirin be? But take it from this doctor: You should resist. Even though aspirin is an over-the-counter drug, it still is a medicine that has potentially serious side effects. To protect your health, never take any drug, even one that seems as innocuous as aspirin, without fully knowing the potential risks. For people at high risk of heart disease or who already have cardiovascular disease, the potential benefits will outweigh the risks—not necessarily so for someone with a different health profile.

To understand the trade-offs, you need to know a bit about why heart attacks and strokes happen and how aspirin works. Heart attacks and strokes can be caused by clots that form in critical arteries and block blood flow. When this happens in an artery supplying blood to your heart, you have a heart attack; when it happens in an artery providing blood to your brain, you have a stroke. Aspirin has a number of actions but works primarily by reducing clot formation in these arteries. It inhibits the actions of platelets, cellular components in your blood that are an important part of clotting. Normally, when there is a nick in a blood vessel, proteins in your blood work together with platelets to plug the leak. When aspirin is in your system, platelets don't stick together as well. This can help prevent heart attacks and strokes because clots not only form in response to nicks in blood vessels; they also occur when blood vessels are damaged by anything, including atherosclerotic plaques seen in people with high cholesterol. This is the good news.

Now for the bad. While no one wants clots to block critical arteries feeding your heart and brain, there are many times that you *do* want clots to form, for instance when you are bleeding. If clots don't form or form slowly, you run the risk of prolonged bleeding. There's also a chance for a "double whammy." Aspirin can irritate your stomach lining, which can *cause* bleeding and then can interfere with the clot-forming to make the bleeding stop. On rare occasions the amount of bleeding in the gastrointestinal tract can be large, even fatal. In addition, bleeding can occur in other places. If clotting is impaired and bleeding occurs in the brain, taking aspirin can actually *cause* a stroke.

So how do you weigh your benefits and risks? If you have had a previous heart attack or a stroke due to a blockage in an artery, most doctors will recommend that you take a daily baby aspirin. The evidence is pretty strong that it can lower your chance of having a recurrent event. It gets murkier if you have never had a problem. A recent study in the *Journal of the American Medical Association* analyzed data from Italy on more than three hundred thousand people taking aspirin to prevent a first heart attack or stroke. They found that the number of cardiovascular events prevented was about the *same* as the number of episodes of major bleeding caused by the aspirin. In light of these risks, the American Heart Association recommends aspirin only for people who are at high risk of having a heart attack. The U.S. Preventive Services Task Force (USPSTF), the government advisory group that looks at this sort of thing, recommends an aspirin for men ages forty-five to seventy-nine and women ages fifty-five to seventy-nine when the potential benefits outweigh the potential harm due to gastrointestinal bleeding.

Right now there is also growing evidence that daily aspirin use reduces both the occurrence of colonic polyps, the precursors to colon cancer, and the occurrence of colon cancer itself. However, the evidence that it actually reduces deaths from colon cancer is more limited, with some studies showing a benefit and others not. In those studies that do show a benefit, the benefit is small. So why the differences in these studies? Well, most polyps do not go on to become cancers, and polyps picked up by routine colon cancer screening can be removed so that they never have a chance to cause a problem. So what if aspirin prevents something that would not have harmed you?

Just as for heart disease and stroke, you have to ask yourself, what is your risk of getting colon cancer compared with the risks from taking an aspirin? The USPSTF reviewed this issue back in 2007. It found that the benefits of daily aspirin use for the prevention of cancer did not outweigh the risks for people with an average chance of developing colon cancer, as well as those with a family history of colon cancer. While there have been quite a number of studies published since 2007, there hasn't been anything that convinces me that routinely taking aspirin for colon cancer prevention makes sense. Better approach: Get regular, recommended colon cancer screenings, such as a colonoscopy. If you have already had colon cancer, you fall into a different risk group altogether.

DR. B'S BOTTOM LINE:

Who could have guessed that a decision about something as seemingly simple as taking a daily aspirin could be so controversial? Bottom line is that aspirin is not for everyone. Even though it's sold over the counter, it is a real drug with real side effects. For those who have had a heart attack in the past, it can really be a lifesaver. However, if you don't need it, don't take it. Before starting on aspirin or any nonprescribed drug, have an open conversation with your doctor about risk, benefit, and how to view the trade-offs.

ASPIRIN TO THE RESCUE

Rosie O'Donnell credits taking an aspirin when she thought she might be having a heart attack with saving her life. If you think you are having a heart attack, first call 911. Then chew an aspirin (preferably one without enteric coating) and wash it down with a glass of water. Chewing it up will help it get absorbed faster and go to work preventing further clot formation.

40

ARE NAME-BRAND DRUGS BETTER THAN GENERIC?

I have to admit it. I am a bit of a brand-name snob. I have my favorite brand of soap, corn flakes, ice cream, sneakers, and jeans. For some reason, I am not very excited about buying store brands for any of these. I guess the marketing has gotten to me. I know what I want—or at least I have been convinced that I do by the millions of dollars in advertisements.

So I'm not surprised that you may be hesitant about giving up your brand-name drug for the generic equivalent. The pharmaceutical industry spends billions of dollars on advertisements every year to build their market and brand loyalty. How can the store version do the same thing as the expensive stuff? It doesn't always look the same. The size and color are different and it may not even the taste the same. How many times have you played mental Ping-Pong, glancing at the side-by-side over-the-counter pain relievers, one brand name, one store brand, wondering whether it's worth paying the extra few dollars for the brand-name version? Surely, there's a reason that the "no-name" box is cheaper. After all, why would anyone pay more for the same product? Turns out, there's no good reason to.

The generic forms of drugs can save you potentially thousands of dollars a year without affecting your health. Here's why. The FDA requires that generic drugs be chemically identical and be as safe and effective as their brand-name counterparts. While they might not look exactly the same, they must have the same active chemicals. The company making the generic drug must do studies to show the FDA that the same amount of the drug gets into your bloodstream, meaning it will work the same.

There is a reason why generic drugs cost so much less than the brand-name ones. When drug companies develop a new product, they bear the costs of years of research and development in order to bring it to market. Because of these huge investments, manufacturers are rewarded with patent protection for twenty years. The patent protects the manufacturer's investment in the drug by giving the manufacturer exclusive rights to sell the drug during the life of the patent. Once the patent expires, other manufacturers can apply to the FDA for approval to market a generic version of the product. These manufacturers don't need to pay for research, development, or marketing, so their costs are much, much lower. When several companies get approval to manufacture generics, competition drives the price down further.

According to the FDA, nearly 80 percent of prescriptions filled in the United States are for generic drugs. That percentage is expected to grow as many popular medications continue to come off patent. In just one year big-ticket drugs including Lipitor for high cholesterol, Plavix for preventing blood clots, Lexapro for depression, and Singulair for asthma went generic.

Surprisingly, brand-name manufacturers frequently make generic versions of their own or other brand-name drugs. For example, Pfizer, the maker of the cholesterol-lowering drug Lipitor, was also the manufacturer of the first generic clone! The manufacturer may also make slight changes in the formulation (how much drug per pill, how a drug is absorbed) as a means of trying to extend their patent protection and safeguard their share of the market. Even after a patent expires, the brand-name manufacturer often continues to advertise their version, hoping you will still perceive its superiority and be willing to pay more for it. There is no legitimacy to this marketing ploy, but like much direct-to-consumer advertising of drugs, it is quite effective.

DR. B'S BOTTOM LINE:

You can feel secure about getting the same quality *and* saving money by buying generic versions of a drug. You'll be getting the same benefits but at less cost.

NOT SO DIFFERENT AFTER ALL

To gain FDA approval, a generic drug must:

- Be identical in strength, dosage form, and route of administration and have the same indications for use.
- Contain the same active ingredients as the innovator drug (inactive ingredients may vary) and reach the same levels in the blood.
- Meet the same batch requirements for identity, strength, purity, and quality.
- Be manufactured under the same strict standards of FDA's good manufacturing practice regulations required for innovator products.

Source: FDA, What Are Generics? www.fda.gov/Drugs/ResourcesForYou/Consumers /BuyingUsingMedicineSafely/UnderstandingGenericDrugs/ucm144456.htm.

41

CAN I USE A DRUG AFTER THE EXPIRATION DATE?

Here's a pop quiz. What do the following have in common: A bad case of poison ivy, the flu, a sprained ankle, and menstrual cramps? Give up? They are all conditions that lead us to buy medications that end up being used a few times before being forgotten and pushed to the back of wherever you keep your drugs, typically the medicine cabinet. As they sit and sit, another thing happens. They pass their expiration dates, leaving you with that big dilemma when you need them again: Do you throw them away and buy new ones, or do you risk it and use them anyway?

This uncertainty is the reason for many after-hours calls. Some patients wonder if the drugs are still effective; others fear they could be dangerous. With food we've been conditioned to think if it's expired, it's time to get rid of it. I don't know anyone who would think of drinking milk two weeks after its stamped date, let alone a year or two! Luckily, there is an extensive body of research looking into the safety of using drugs after their expiration dates. It agrees that, in most cases, prescription and over-the-counter drugs remain safe and effective *long* after those printed dates.

Here's why. To protect the public, beginning in 1979 drug companies were legally required to put a date that their drug would still be *good* on the package. Herein lies the major distinction: The FDA did not require a date to indicate when the drug would theoretically start to "go bad," nor did it require drug companies to test for that. The drug companies just needed to provide a date for which they would guarantee that the medication would still be *good*. For most drugs, the pharmaceutical companies assigned a relatively arbitrary and short time frame—generally two to three years. Manufacturers claimed that the longer they needed to keep drugs on hand to continue to test their efficacy, the more costs they would have to pass on to consumers. Given this, they chose very conservative dates for expiration.

This subject of drug longevity is one I know well. For four of the years I worked at the CDC, I was responsible for the Strategic National Stockpile. Few people realize that the government has amassed a huge collection of critical antibiotics, vaccines, and other drugs to be used in the event of public health emergencies. We've been lucky and most haven't been needed, so they sit in waiting. The drugs in the stockpile are worth billions of dollars, so the government does not want to discard them unless it has to. As part of our country's Shelf Life Extension Program, drugs are periodically tested for potency and safety. These tests have shown that most of the drugs remain effective for many years longer than would be expected based on expiration dates.

The general public's knowledge of this program's findings is very limited. I found this out firsthand when I went knocking on doors and looking into people's medicine cabinets for a "Doc at the Door" segment on *Good Morning America*. Let me tell you, you really get to know someone after seeing what's in his medicine cabinet! There was one thing all the people I spoke to had in common. They were all unsure how to manage their medicines, and much of their confusion stemmed from not knowing when to keep and when to discard prescription and over-the-counter medications.

Drug companies are in business to make money. It's in their best interest for you to frequently replenish medications, even when they are still effective. When it comes to deciding what to use and what not to use after the expiration date, here's my advice:

- For critical medications (heart drugs, blood pressure medications, etc.) stick to the expiration dates. If you are being prescribed correctly, you shouldn't come near to approaching the typical one-year date.
- For non-liquid over-the-counter medications being stored in a cool, dark place, don't worry about the expiration dates.
- For antibiotics, it's a good idea to stick to the expiration date, too. Some antibiotics lose potency over time or if improperly stored. When

prescribed a course of antibiotics, finish them! If you have an old container of antibiotics, get rid of them properly. If you are given antibiotics to use sporadically for prevention of a urinary tract infection, discard them when they reach the expiration date.

- For liquids, I'd stick close to the expiration date. They tend to degrade faster than pills.
- For all medications, if the appearance or the smell of the medicine has changed, throw it out.

DR. B'S BOTTOM LINE:

This issue is so confusing, it's enough to give you a headache. We have been conditioned to believe that "expiration date" actually means the date after which something is no longer good. Fortunately, for most drugs, that is not the case. Their expiration dates only guarantee that a medication is good on that date, even if it's just as likely to still be effective five years past that date. Unless the regulations on this change (and I see nothing to suggest that they will), you need to follow your personal risk tolerance. But I bet if you follow my simple rules, you will be making fewer late-night trips to the drugstore.

HELP KEEP YOUR WATER SUPPLY SAFE

Prevent medication from getting into the water system. Dispose of medications using this simple method: Mix pills in a sealable plastic bag with a little water and coffee grounds or kitty litter so they dissolve, and then throw the sealed bag in the trash.

42

ARE OVER-THE-COUNTER PAIN RELIEVERS INTERCHANGEABLE?

When my wife has a headache or a fever, she always says, "I'm going to take some aspirin." She doesn't mean she is actually going to take an aspirin. It is just the word she and many other people use for a pain or fever reliever. When we were kids that was what we took. Now there are choices. Acetaminophen (Tylenol and generics) gained popularity throughout the 1960s and ibuprofen (Motrin, Advil, and generics) became available over the counter in 1984.

So when you have a headache, fever, or aches and pains, which one do you take and does it matter? Are all pain and fever relievers equal?

They are not. Each drug works in a different way and has different strengths and side effects that you need to know about. If you learn the basics, it's easy to reach for the right one for what ails you. If you're treating a particular medical condition, like arthritis or migraines, have your doctor go over them with you to see what will be best for you.

Here are the basics:

Aspirin: Aspirin is a member of a class of drugs called nonsteroidal anti-inflammatory drugs, or NSAIDs. These drugs work in part by blocking the production of prostaglandins, chemicals in your body that regulate inflammation, fever, and pain. Aspirin is also used for the prevention of heart disease in high-risk people and in the treatment of heart attacks, strokes, and a number of joint disorders. Like all drugs in this class, it can cause indigestion, heartburn, and ulcers. Because aspirin has been linked to Reye's syndrome, a serious and sometimes fatal illness in children, it shouldn't be given to any child younger than nineteen years old unless directed to by a doctor. Another caution: Aspirin interferes with how your blood clots. That makes it good for preventing clotting in your heart vessels, but dangerous if you are prone to bleeding.

Ibuprofen: Like aspirin, ibuprofen is also an NSAID. It is very useful for treating muscle pain, body aches, and fever and is often used for menstrual cramps. NSAIDs are quite safe when used for short periods of time, but extended use has been linked to an increased risk of stomach bleeding, heart attack, stroke, and kidney failure. It's best to take this drug after you've had something to eat to reduce any stomach distress. As with any NSAID, don't take it for more than ten days without checking with your doctor.

Acetaminophen: Like ibuprofen, acetaminophen lowers fever and reduces pain. However, it is not an NSAID and doesn't reduce inflammation, so is not recommended for body aches and pains from overworked muscles. What I really like about this drug is that it is easy on the stomach, so it does not need to be taken with food. There's a big warning with acetaminophen, though. In large doses it is very toxic to the liver. For adults, never take more than 3,000 mg (3 grams) in a single day. It actually is pretty easy to reach this limit. Extra-strength products contain 500 mg per tablet or capsule, so if you take two every six hours, you will reach the limit. You have to be very careful because quite a number of over-the-counter cold, flu, and sleep products also contain acetaminophen in combination with other drugs. Because of this, always read the label to make sure you aren't taking in too much. Another caveat: If you have liver disease or have more than three drinks per day, stay away from this drug!

Generally, my advice for adults relates to preference. Over time you may find that you tolerate or get relief from one of these drugs more than the others. If you have any medical conditions, talk to your doctor about which medication is best for you. For example, ibuprofen can interfere with the heart-protective benefits of aspirin.

Here's a brief recommendation and overview by symptom.

Fever: Acetaminophen or ibuprofen. One advantage of ibuprofen is that the dosing is every eight hours versus every six hours for acetaminophen. A number of systematic reviews in children show a benefit of ibuprofen over acetaminophen for fever relief.

Headache: Acetaminophen or ibuprofen. I like the side-effect profile of acetaminophen better than for the NSAIDs as long as you pay attention to the dose. Otherwise either of these is fine. There are some studies that show that caffeine adds to the relief from these drugs. I'd be careful, though, since caffeine withdrawal is also a cause of headaches.

Muscle aches and pains, menstrual cramps: Ibuprofen. The anti-inflammatory properties of this drug make it my favorite.

Hangover: Ibuprofen or aspirin. Remember that acetaminophen is toxic to the liver. If you've been drinking too much, give your liver a break and use one of these other drugs.

DR. B'S BOTTOM LINE:

Pain and fever relievers are not created equal. Know the side effects and the benefits of each. Also make sure to use caution when using them with other over-the-counter multipurpose medications to make sure you aren't taking more than the daily recommended dose. Even though these are not prescription drugs, there are risks from taking too much of them.

43

ARE HERBAL SUPPLEMENTS AS EFFECTIVE AS OTHER MEDICATIONS?

Walk through any health food store and you'll see shelves lined with various herbal supplements. We've all heard the claims: Echinacea supports your immune system, gingko improves memory, raspberry ketones help you lose weight. In my clinical practice, I always get questions about "natural" supplements. I get it. We all want to feel better when we're sick and want to prevent illness. There's always a friend who doesn't trust conventional medicine and is suspicious of the pharmaceutical industry but swears by something alternative. Plus, there's comfort in the word *herbal*. After all, aren't herbal remedies natural? That should make them safe and good for you, shouldn't it?

When it comes to herbal supplements, safe is not something that should come to mind. In fact, to me, herbal supplements are some of the scariest remedies out there because they are, in essence, self-regulated.

I don't have anything against looking to nature for cures. Many drugs used in conventional medicine are derived from plants and herbs. However, before these drugs are marketed, pharmaceutical companies are required to do safety studies and conduct clinical trials to show that they are effective. As a doctor and scientist, that just makes sense to me. Look to the natural world for potential treatments, then assess them scientifically for effectiveness. I wish that were true for supplements.

When you take an herbal supplement or remedy, you have *no* way of knowing what the active (druglike) ingredients are or whether the amount contained in two similar products is the same. You have no way of knowing whether the claims on the label have been tested and proven, unlike when you take a prescribed drug that meets FDA standards.

Shocked? I was when I first started looking into this. The most incredible thing to me is that this was a deliberate decision by Congress. In 1994, they basically said to the FDA, the agency entrusted with ensuring a safe and effective drug supply, "hands off the vitamin and supplement industry." They passed the Dietary Supplement Health and Education Act (DSHEA). This legislation placed dietary supplements in a special category under the general umbrella of "foods" instead. Under the DSHEA, the manufacturer became responsible for ensuring that its products are safe before they are marketed. According to the FDA, "Unlike drug products that must be proven safe and effective for their intended use before marketing, there are no provisions in the law for FDA to 'approve' dietary supplements for safety or effectiveness before they reach the consumer." The FDA adds, "Unlike drugs, supplements *are not intended to treat, diagnose, prevent, or cure diseases*." That means supplements cannot make claims, such as "reduces arthritic pain" or "treats heart disease." Per the FDA, these claims can only legitimately be made for drugs.

Surprised? That is because the advertising for supplements frequently walks a fine line. A supplement can purport to support a strong immune system rather than claim to prevent colds. It can claim to promote weight loss rather than to treat obesity. Pick up any supplement and you will see an asterisk on the label. If you have really good vision you will read the tiny disclaimer that says that the claims on the label "have not been evaluated by the FDA."

To add insult to injury, under DSHEA, once the product is marketed, the FDA has to *prove* that a dietary supplement is "unsafe" before it can take action to restrict the product's use or force its removal from the marketplace. Talk about a sweet deal! Supplements are a multibillion-dollar business. Whose lawyers do you think are going to win most of those fights? Manufacturers are entrusted to "verify" that their products are safe and not make any misleading claims about their medical benefits.

Let's look at the über-popular herbal supplement Airborne, marketed to prevent colds. In 2008, it had to shell out over $23 million to settle a class-action lawsuit brought against the company for false advertising. A report on *Good Morning America* revealed that what Airborne claimed was a double-blind, placebo-controlled study by a company specializing in clinical trial management was really conducted by two guys with no medical degrees. The company ceased referring to its product as a cold remedy and removed those claims from the box, now choosing to say it can help support your immune system. Somehow I don't think it is the only supplement manufacturer that might have fudged a thing or two.

Echinacea, another popular herbal remedy touted for preventing and treating colds, has also shown inconsistent scientific basis for those claims. A 2005 study in the *New England Journal of Medicine* found no benefits from echinacea for rhinovirus (colds) over placebo. In 2009, Cochrane, an independent health care review system, examined sixteen controlled clinical trials comparing different echinacea preparations for preventing and treating common colds. There was no evidence that it prevented colds. Other studies looked at whether it shortened the duration or decreased the severity of the symptoms once a cold was contracted compared with a placebo. Some studies showed that preparations based on the herb of *Echinacea purpurea* might provide some benefits for cold relief in adults, but none in children. The problem with relying too much on these results is the inconsistency from product to product. Various supplement manufacturers use different species of the herb, different parts of the plant, and different manufacturing processes, so any potential benefits could differ from one brand to another.

So what should you do if you use supplements? The first thing is to find out if what you are using is safe. Some supplements can increase or decrease the effectiveness of medications you are currently taking. Talk to your doctor about this. In the meantime, visit the NIH website on Complementary and Alternative Medicine. There you will find great information on the effectiveness of supplements and potential dangers. As a physician, I want to see scientific evidence before I recommend anything to my patients. You should demand the same standards for any product you put in your body.

DR. B'S BOTTOM LINE:

Buyer beware! Being dependent on supplements isn't good for your health or your pocketbook. Most herbal supplements have not been tested scientifically to see if they work and the claims you see on the label have not been independently evaluated. Just because something is "natural" does not mean it is safe.

44

WHAT ARE THE MOST DANGEROUS DRUGS?

Picture this: A back alley, a junkie slumped over behind a Dumpster, dead from heroin. That is the image of a drug overdose that I, and I think many others, have from movies and news reports. However, the rising problem of drug abuse looks much different from what we might expect. Instead of strung-out addicts, think soccer moms, colleagues at work, and high school and college students. Think about legal prescription drugs. The United States is facing an *epidemic* of prescription pain medication abuse. In 2007, prescription narcotic painkillers were involved in more unintentional overdose deaths than heroin and cocaine combined! Even more disturbing, in 2009, for the first time in the thirty years that the government has been tracking drug-induced deaths, drug overdoses and the effects of long-term drug abuse killed more people than motor vehicle accidents.

It might start innocently enough, with nagging back pain that keeps you from getting to work. Maybe it's insomnia that you can't seem to beat. Or you just need a little oomph to get that big project done. One or two pills turn into a few more, and before you realize it, you can't get through the day or night without them. Drugs commonly involved in unintentional deaths include pain relievers, tranquilizers, antidepressants, stimulants, and sedatives. You may recognize the names: OxyContin, Vicodin, Xanax, all commonly abused, highly addictive prescription drugs.

This epidemic affects all ages. The National Institute on Drug Abuse (NIDA) reported that in 2009, sixteen million Americans ages twelve and older had taken a prescription pain reliever, tranquilizer, stimulant, or sedative for nonmedical purposes at least once in the year prior to being surveyed. For many, use begins in high school. As teens become adults, the rates continue to rise. While we tend to think of drug abuse and overdose as the plague of youth, the forty-five-to-fifty-four-year-old age group had the highest rate of unintentional drug overdoses.

Why is prescription drug abuse so common? Largely because the use of these drugs does not carry the same stigma as the use of illicit drugs. Many people feel that because doctors prescribe them, they must be safe to take. And once you have a prescription drug problem, getting drugs isn't hard. More than half of all prescription drug users get them from family and friends, *not* physicians. Others learn how to scam the system to get drugs. It can be very difficult for doctors to tell whether a patient has significant pain for which a narcotic pain reliever might be warranted or is just trying to get drugs. Many doctors are undertrained in pain management or don't take the time to prescribe properly.

Prescription drugs aren't the only problem. Just because you don't need a prescription for over-the-counter (OTC) painkillers, it doesn't mean they are universally safe. While OTC painkillers like acetaminophen (Tylenol), aspirin, and ibuprofen (Motrin) lack the addictive potential of powerful prescription pain medications, they pose serious health risks if misused. An unintentional overdose of acetaminophen can seriously damage your liver and even cause death.

Pain relievers are commonly found in other medications as well, making it easy to ingest more than intended. Acetaminophen poisoning is now the most common cause of acute liver failure in the United States. The risk of overdose has become so significant that companies such as Johnson & Johnson, makers of Tylenol, reduced the recommended daily dose from eight pills (4,000 mg) to six pills (3,000 mg) to protect users from accidental overdoses. Ten thousand milligrams can destroy your liver.

Take this example, which shows how easy it can be to get into trouble: You have the flu and feel achy, feverish, and congested. You wake up feeling terrible so you pop two extra-strength acetaminophen tablets for pain relief. That's 1,000 mg. The package says you can take six tablets over the course of the day, which you eagerly do, for a total of 3,000 mg. You also take an OTC multisymptom cold and flu medication, such as Dayquil, to help with the congestion and flu symptoms. This product also contains acetaminophen. The instructions say you can take four doses in twenty-four hours, so over the course of the day you take a total of eight tablets.

That's another 2,600 mg of acetaminophen. Then to help you sleep, you take NyQuil. One dose contains 650 mg of acetaminophen. You might not realize it, but by simply taking common cold and fever medications, you have consumed almost 7,000 mg of acetaminophen. This is more than twice what is recommended and for some, could be a toxic dose. When you're feeling bad as it is, you may not think to calculate all the milligrams you've taken over the day, but they keep adding up. Acetaminophen is even found in prescription painkillers, such as Percocet and Vicodin. If you start with acetaminophen to control your discomfort and end up taking something stronger because you still need relief, you could be setting yourself up for trouble.

Now is also a good time to go through your medicine cabinet and make sure you don't unintentionally become someone's drug supplier. When I was in my thirties, I had multiple episodes of severe back pain, which finally led me to have surgery. Over the course of five years I was prescribed muscle relaxants and narcotic pain pills. When one drug wouldn't work, I would get a stronger one. Over the years, I built up quite a pharmacy in my closet, loaded with addictive and potentially dangerous drugs. It wasn't until I had someone coming to stay with us who I knew had a prescription drug problem that I went through my medications and discarded them properly. Don't wait until it is too late. Take a look—you may be surprised at what you find.

DR. B'S BOTTOM LINE:

Addiction and deaths from prescription pain relievers are skyrocketing. Occasional use can lead to dependence and addiction. Never take medication that has not been prescribed for you and make sure you understand how to take your medications safely. Use caution when using OTC medications as well. Always know what is in the medicines you are taking, and be aware of the safe limits for these drugs. They can also be deadly.

THINGS YOU CAN DO TO KEEP "DRUG SAFE"

- Ask your doctor how to safely use any medication, especially ones for pain, sedation, or anxiety. Ask if it can be addicting or produce unwanted side effects. Be specific on how much you should take and how long you should use it before you should be seen again.
- Make your doctor spend time with you. Don't be afraid to explore other routes to go beyond pills that can be addicting. Rushed doctors are often more likely to write a prescription than to spend the time trying to explore other options.
- Explore alternative therapies with a professional. If you have trouble sleeping, instead of asking for sleeping pills, talk through your sleep habits, explore relaxation techniques, and inquire about nonaddictive medications.
- Be realistic about your discomfort. Doctors are more sympathetic to pain and might try to manage it more aggressively than in the past. Don't exaggerate your symptoms for sympathy or to justify needing to see your doctor. Sometimes an over-the-counter medication is just as appropriate for moderate pain.
- Keep all medication out of the reach of children. Make sure all drugs have childproof tops and are properly closed. Best to not let little children see you taking pills. They love to copy what their parents do.
- Know yourself. If you have an addictive personality, a problem with painkillers, or low pain threshold, let the doctor know about it before he or she prescribes.
- Check all multisymptom medications and highlight the painkiller contained in each to make it easier to track total consumption.

45

SHOULD I TAKE A STATIN TO PREVENT HIGH CHOLESTEROL?

One of our good friends, Don, is the picture of health. Although he just celebrated his sixtieth birthday, he barely looks a day over forty. It's no wonder; playing competitive ice hockey several times a week for decades has left him slim and fit. Looking at him, few could imagine Don's been fighting high cholesterol and heart disease for much of his life. He's not alone. Today, the most common cause of death in America for *both* men and women is heart disease. Of the many risk factors, one of the most important is high cholesterol.

So where does most of this cholesterol come from? Surprisingly, it's not from your diet. Your body manufactures cholesterol and uses it widely: To form the walls of your cells; to produce the hormones that send signals throughout your body, including vitamin D, estrogen, and testosterone; and to help you digest your food. You could not live without cholesterol. The amount of cholesterol measured in your blood is a balance between what you make, what you eat, and what you get rid of. High-density lipoprotein (HDL), also known as good cholesterol, is involved in transporting cholesterol back to your liver for elimination. It is a good marker for how well you get rid of cholesterol. Low-density lipoprotein (LDL), also known as bad cholesterol, is linked to a buildup of cholesterol in your blood and the formation of plaques in your arteries. These plaques—a combination of cholesterol, calcium, platelets, and other material—can block your arteries and cause a heart attack or stroke. A high blood level of LDL cholesterol is a risk factor for heart disease, whereas a high level of HDL cholesterol is a marker for protection from heart disease.

There has been much interest in drugs that can lower your LDL cholesterol, as well as those that can raise your HDL cholesterol. So far, drug therapy to raise your HDL cholesterol has not been very promising. Drugs that have been able to do so haven't been shown to reduce the risk of heart disease or save lives. It is a different story for statins, drugs that reduce

LDL cholesterol. Statins block the production of cholesterol and may even help reabsorb cholesterol in plaques that have already formed. For people who have heart disease or who are at great risk of having a heart attack, statins are an important treatment tool. The popularity of these drugs is almost unrivaled; millions of Americans take them daily. That includes Don, whose father died from heart disease at a young age and who is genetically disposed to having high cholesterol, which can't be controlled through exercise or diet. For Don and others like him, it's amazing how well they work. But for others whose situations are less definitive, whether to automatically use statins is less clear. Sure, they can lower LDL cholesterol in anyone, but is that necessarily the way to go?

Let's look at my wife, Jeanne, for example. She follows all the rules: Rarely eats high saturated-fat foods, exercises almost every day, and has never smoked. However, she also has a family history of high cholesterol. No matter what she does in terms of diet and exercise, her body keeps her LDL and total cholesterol a little on the high side. Fortunately, she also has a high level of HDL cholesterol. I was curious to see if she might benefit from a statin. This year after she got her results from her blood work, I sat down and calculated her risk for heart disease. You should do it, too, using this tool: www.nhlbi.nih.gov/guidelines/cholesterol/atglance.htm.

There's a list of risk factors: First, do you already have atherosclerotic disease (plaques in your arteries)? This could include a history of angina (chest pain), blockages in the arteries in your neck, or poor circulation to your hands and feet. For my wife the answer was a resounding "no" to all of these. Second, if you don't already have diseased arteries, do you have big risk factors for heart disease such as: Smoking, high blood pressure, low HDL cholesterol, a family history of early heart disease (in a male, close relative under fifty-five years; in a female, close relative under sixty-five years), and age (if you are a man, are you over forty-five years; if a woman, over fifty-five years)? Again, for Jeanne, the answers were no to all of these. Next, I used a special calculator to predict her risk of having a heart attack or dying from heart disease within the next ten years. This is called your Framingham Risk Score (hp2010.nhlbihin.net/atpIII/calculator.asp?usertype=prof). I know this sounds complicated, but if you try it, you'll see it isn't.

Using this tool, Jeanne's ten-year risk of having a heart attack or dying of heart disease is only 1 percent, *even* with her elevated cholesterol levels. In cases like Jeanne's, you should weigh the benefits of statins against the possible side effects. Although a statin might lower that risk of heart disease even further, when the potential benefits of a treatment are small, you really need to look at risks. For statins, the side effects are rare but include muscle pain or inflammation, confusion, and an increased risk of developing diabetes. If you truly have heart disease or are at great risk for heart disease, the benefits of the drug would likely outweigh these risks. However, if you are at low risk for heart disease to begin with, why take a drug for the rest of your life that could have any potential side effects?

One more point about statins bears mentioning because you may hear a lot about it. There is mounting evidence that among the main benefits of statin therapy is not just the reduction in bad cholesterol, it is its role in reducing inflammation in your blood vessels. Inflammation in your blood vessels creates a setting for plaque to form. If you reduce inflammation, there will be less plaque. Less plaque means fewer blockages of your arteries. This may help to explain why in some studies, statins reduce the risk of heart disease even in patients who don't have very high cholesterol. Inflammation can be measured by a blood test called the C-reactive protein and more doctors are checking this as well, as a means to prevent heart disease. By the way, Jeanne had hers measured, too—it was also low. By either approach, standard heart disease risk or inflammation, the balance for her and for many others with elevated cholesterol levels would not support taking a statin.

DR. B'S BOTTOM LINE:

Statins are not for everyone. While the benefits of statins may seem like a slam dunk, particularly considering the high prevalence of heart-related deaths,

there is still considerable controversy over whether they are suitable for all people regardless of heart disease risk. If you are at high risk of dying of heart disease or stroke, then there is great benefit in taking a medicine that significantly lowers that risk. If you are not at great risk of dying from heart attack or stroke, who cares if a drug lowers your cholesterol and risk even further?

THINKING BEYOND THE PILL

Some patients can manage their cholesterol without medications. Regardless of whether you end up taking a drug, these measures will reduce your overall risk of heart disease.

- Eat a heart-healthy diet:
  - Low in saturated and trans fats and cholesterol: Make it a turkey burger and hold the cheese. While you are at it, ask for extra veggies and a whole wheat bun.
  - High in fiber: Start your day with oatmeal or high-fiber cereal topped with fruit. Make your own granola (to help control the amount of oil and sweeteners) and add bran and dried fruit.
- Keep the extra pounds off. If you are overweight, losing the extra pounds can bring down your cholesterol.
- Move it. Regular exercise can lower your cholesterol.
- Quit smoking. This won't reduce your cholesterol but it will limit the damage to your blood vessels that allows cholesterol-laden plaques to form.

46

SHOULD I USE HORMONE THERAPY FOR MY MENOPAUSE SYMPTOMS?

It is hard to think of a class of medications that has a more checkered and disturbing history than hormone therapy in women. Beginning in the 1960s estrogens and then combination estrogen and progesterone products were marketed to women to treat the symptoms of menopause—then considered a disease—and to prevent its alleged consequences: heart disease, Alzheimer's disease, and osteoporosis.

Never has a drug seen such widespread acceptance based on such flimsy medical evidence. It wasn't until high-quality randomized, double-blinded controlled trials were conducted that the truth became known. For most women, the risks from using menopausal hormone therapy far outweighed the benefits.

As anyone who has lived through or lived with someone going through menopause knows, it's not easy. As levels of estrogen and progesterone decrease, the body goes through a multitude of unpleasant changes. For many women—and for many years—hormone therapy (formerly called hormone replacement therapy) was a godsend when it came to dealing with the unwelcome side effects of menopause.

Generally speaking, hormone therapy involves artificial supplementation with hormones that decline at the time of menopause. In addition to addressing bothersome hot flashes and night sweats—two of the most common complaints associated with menopause—hormone therapy also deals with some of the vaginal symptoms of menopause, such as dryness and itching, and may reduce the risk for hip fractures.

Initial studies found other benefits. Women who took hormone therapy were less likely to develop heart disease and dementia. However, these studies were quite misleading. Women were not randomly assigned to take these drugs; instead researchers looked at the outcomes for women who chose to take them and compared them to women who chose not to.

In the case of hormone therapy, prescribing information for some products indicated that women with heart disease should not take them. It was no surprise, therefore, that fewer women taking the drugs had heart disease.

It wasn't until randomized controlled trials were conducted that the truth was shown. The Women's Health Initiative study, or WHI for short, is perhaps the most well known study to reveal these risks. This study enrolled more than 160,000 postmenopausal women between fifty and seventy-nine years of age between 1993 and 1998 and was designed to quantify the benefits of hormone therapy in the realm of cardiovascular disease.

Instead the WHI study delivered a devastating one-two punch to hormone therapy. Not only was the risk of coronary heart disease found to be 29 percent higher in women taking hormone therapy when compared to the placebo group; the risk of breast cancer was 26 percent higher in women taking the medication. Only modest reductions were seen in the rates of colorectal cancer and hip fractures in women taking hormone therapy— not nearly enough to offset the harm.

Despite this large-scale study and later ones that have similar findings, the debate over whether hormone therapy increases the risk of chronic disease continues. Some are looking to see if there are subgroups of women for whom the drugs are safe and effective. Others call into question the methods used in the large controlled drug trials.

The U.S. Preventive Services Task Force (USPSTF) has issued recommendations that are quite clear. They recommend against the use of hormone therapy for the prevention of chronic disease of any kind, including heart disease or fractures. They found that while hormone therapy decreased the risk of fractures and colon cancer, it increased the risk of stroke, gallbladder disease, urinary incontinence, dementia, blood clots, and breast cancer. The trade-off was just not worth it. This is in keeping with the recommendations of many other medical societies. The USPSTF did not address the use of hormone therapy for treating severe menopausal symptoms.

Many women continue to take these drugs despite studies that suggest health risks, primarily because they see these drugs as their best option for dealing with severe symptoms of menopause. The FDA still approves of the use of hormone therapy for treating menopausal symptoms and for the prevention of osteoporosis. However, the agency recommends that they be used at the lowest effective dose and for as short a period as possible.

DR. B'S BOTTOM LINE:

The weight of the evidence overwhelmingly demonstrates that hormone therapy poses health risks to postmenopausal women and should not be used for the prevention of any chronic disease. Women with severe menopausal symptoms should ask their doctor about other options for relief, such as low-dose estrogen creams for vaginal symptoms. Some women find they can control some symptoms through yoga and other relaxation techniques. Dressing in layers and keeping your bedroom cool can help with hot flashes. If you can't find comfort any other way, use hormone therapy as briefly as you can.

47

SHOULD I TAKE CALCIUM FOR STRONG BONES?

You've all heard the adage "A picture is worth a thousand words." Nowhere is that more true than the ubiquitous "Got Milk" campaign. Seeing the thin, white mustache above a celebrity's mouth symbolizes the benefits of drinking milk. For most people that means recognizing the importance of calcium in your diet.

Calcium is a critical component of our bones and is very important for bone strength. Vitamin D is an important regulator of calcium absorption from the intestine. In growing bones, extreme deficiencies of calcium and vitamin D can lead to rickets. In adults it can cause bone demineralization and, in some people, osteoporosis.

Osteoporosis is a condition marked by severe thinning of the bones and an increased risk for fractures. It is seen primarily in elderly postmenopausal women. Roughly one-half of all postmenopausal women will have a fracture due to osteoporosis at some point in their lives. The big fracture everyone worries about is of the hip. For older women and men, a hip fracture can be a life-altering and life-ending experience. It is an event that can render previously active people immobile for months, and it can impact their quality of life forever. A third of men who have a hip fracture are dead within a year.

Conventional wisdom would suggest that, if your bones are brittle from too little mineralization, increasing the intake of calcium would help. This principle, in fact, is the basis for the massive sale of calcium supplements—one of the most popular on the market today. According to the CDC, 61 percent of women older than sixty take calcium supplements. Unfortunately, the evidence is pretty inconclusive that taking calcium and vitamin D supplements leads to improved bone health. The USPSTF has suggested that, for now at least, the evidence is too shaky to recommend the use of calcium supplements, with or without vitamin D. A review of the randomized controlled trials found little benefit, though the quality of studies in terms of the amount and types of supplements used varied. They concluded that daily supplementation with 400 IU (international units) of vitamin D and 1,000 mg of calcium did not reduce fractures due to osteoporosis.

America's love affair with calcium supplementation is emblematic of its love affair with supplements in general. Many people accept on faith that supplements will improve health. More often when formal studies are done, supplements have been shown to cause harm. Getting too much calcium increases your risk of kidney stones—not a large increase in risk, but an increase nonetheless. More concerning are several studies linking calcium supplementation to a small but real increase in heart attacks and strokes. The theory is that taking large doses of calcium leads to the calcium being deposited not just in your bones, but also in the plaques that are forming in your coronary arteries. The larger the plaque, the more likely it is to block blood flow to your heart and brain. Unlike dietary calcium, which is absorbed slowly, supplements give your body a large amount of calcium all at once.

The better approach is to get the calcium you need from your diet throughout the day, to allow it to be absorbed slowly. The National Osteoporosis Foundation (NOF), an industry-supported advocacy group, also endorses food as the best source of calcium. Eating a diet that includes dairy products and leafy green vegetables, in addition to calcium-fortified foods, easily allows you to reach your daily goals. The Institute of Medicine has laid out recommendations for calcium intake. For healthy adults, the recommended intake is 1,000 to 1,200 mg per day. With a little bit of planning, it isn't that hard to do. Foods rich in calcium include low-fat or nonfat milk, yogurt, cheese, sardines, salmon, broccoli, and dark leafy vegetables such as kale, in addition to calcium-fortified orange juice and cereals. Start your day with a combination of these foods and you'll quickly be at your recommended intake. The NOF also cautions against getting more calcium than you need through supplements, citing the lack of any additional benefits and warning of possible risks.

DR. B'S BOTTOM LINE:

When it comes to preventing weakened bones, calcium supplementation may not be as useful as you think. Try to get the calcium you need from your diet. It isn't the same as getting it through pills.

STRONG BONES, HEALTHY BONES

While you're thinking about your bones, make sure you don't ignore other risk factors for osteoporosis, and make those little changes that can make a big difference. The USPSTF recommends that women who are older than sixty-five, and younger women with risk factors for bone loss, get screened for osteoporosis. The approach to treatment at that point depends on your ten-year risk for having a hip fracture or other significant fracture. You can calculate your risk online using FRAX, the World Health Organization Fracture Risk Assessment Tool (www.shef.ac.uk/FRAX/tool.jsp?country=9)

Your goal in terms of bone health is to do what you can to maintain strong ones. This applies to everyone, regardless of age. There are a number of risk factors for osteoporosis to be aware of because many can be changed. If any characteristics on the following list apply to you, be sure to get adequate calcium in your diet by eating dairy- and calcium-enriched foods. But don't stop there. Make an effort to incorporate weight-bearing exercise, including lifting weights or yoga, to strengthen your bones.

- Age: Women over sixty-five years; men over seventy years
- Size: being small and thin
- Taking certain medications including steroids
- Cigarette smoking
- Excessive alcohol consumption
- Lack of exercise

48

WHERE SHOULD I STORE MEDICATIONS?

I bet if I asked a roomful of people where they stored their medicine, 99 percent, if not more, would say in the bathroom medicine cabinet. After all, that's what it's for, isn't it? I actually turned this question around and sprung it on unsuspecting residents in a northern New Jersey neighborhood for a "Doc at your Door" segment. Going door to door, I asked them if I could look in their medicine cabinets—in the name of better health. They were all overflowing with medications. Every single person was shocked when I said that the bathroom is the *worst* place to store both prescription and over-the-counter drugs.

Of all the rooms in your house, the bathroom is the most hot and humid. Just picture a typical morning: Steamy showers, warm water fogging up your bathroom mirror as you shave. Guess what makes medications disintegrate and lose their effectiveness the fastest? Excessive moisture and heat! We all put medicine there but we shouldn't. To protect your drugs' efficacy and longevity, they should be stored in a cool, dry place away from bright light. The back of a linen cabinet, a bedroom shelf, or a kitchen cabinet (away from the sink, stove, and direct sunlight) are all better suited. I like to organize mine in Tupperware-type boxes so I can easily pull them out to find what I'm looking for.

No matter where you decide to house them, make sure all medication is kept out of the reach of children or in a locked cabinet. According to the CDC, each year more than seventy thousand children are seen in the emergency room due to unintentional poisonings. More than 80 percent of the cases involved unsupervised children getting into medicines. Even vitamins, which children confuse with candy, should be kept in a safe place where they can't access them.

This is especially important when you are visiting others. One of the riskiest situations for young children happens every holiday season when Grandma and Grandpa come to visit. Often elderly people keep their medications in pill organizers. These are great tools to help you to remember to take your medications and they are easy to open, which for people with arthritis can be a real benefit. However, if little kids are around, these pill organizers can be deadly. To see for myself how risky this could be, I conducted a totally unscientific experiment for *Good Morning America*. I assembled a group of six incredibly adorable children, two to four years old. First I gave them a variety of pill organizers and asked them to show me how fast they could open them. All six got them open; one three-year-old little girl had hers open in just ten seconds. Next I gave them easy-open prescription bottles like the kind often given to the elderly. Four out of the six kids got into these in less than thirty seconds. Finally, I gave them each a child-resistant pill container. None of the children could open it.

The lessons are clear. Even if your own children are out of the house, when grandchildren or visitors come, make sure to safely store your and their medication out of sight. If you use easy-open pill containers, remember that these can be incredibly dangerous around children. For your everyday medications: Keep them cool, keep them dark, and keep them all locked up.

DR. B'S BOTTOM LINE:

It seems like the bathroom is the most practical place to keep medications, since we often take them when we wake up or before bed, but dry, cool areas really are the best place to store them. Use bathroom cabinets for first aid items and health and beauty supplies that are not affected by heat and moisture. Most importantly, keep all medications out of the reach of children, whether you are at home or visiting.

KEEP YOUR HOUSE SAFE

- Keep all medications in a cool, dark place.
- Don't keep medicine in the refrigerator unless specifically instructed to do so.
- If you have kids in the house, make sure your guests keep medication out of reach and out of sight.
- Make sure the safety cap is sealed on all medications.
- Talk to your kids about the dangers of taking medicine and vitamins without supervision.
- Have the number for poison control handy in case of an emergency: 800-222-1222.
- Prescription drug abuse is on the rise. Beware of leaving prescription painkillers, sedatives, and anti-anxiety medications where someone can get them.

5

AN OUNCE OF PREVENTION, A POUND OF CURE

Your Questions About Understanding, Preventing, and Responding to Illness and Injury

Let's say you've taken important steps toward improving your health. You are trying to eat better, move more, and own your health. You are on the road to a longer, healthier life. Great! Your odds of getting sick have gone way down. However, not everything can be prevented. There are still some medical land mines out there that you need to know about.

For serious conditions including heart attacks, cancer, and stroke, knowing your own risk and familiarizing yourself with symptoms can literally save your life. For less serious but life-disrupting conditions like common infections and back pain, understanding how to avoid or manage them can help to make sure that you are sidelined for as short a time as possible. Here we'll take a closer look at the factors that contribute to both life-threatening diseases and everyday ills, so you can try to prevent them— and know what actions you can take if prevention fails.

For many diseases there is a gender gap. For example, heart disease doesn't always look the same in men and women. Accordingly, treatment isn't provided in the same manner. If you don't know what to look for, how can you get the care you may need?

There are also a number of misconceptions out there. Do you believe that breast cancer is the leading cause of death in women? It's not even close! Find out what is so you can work to prevent that, too.

The truth is, disease is a part of life. But for many maladies, understanding illness and learning how to protect yourself can help prevent more serious consequences and help you recover more quickly.

49

CAN I CATCH THE SAME INFECTION TWICE?

When my son Alex was in fourth grade he had the nicest school nurse ever. Mollie was quickly able to figure out which kids were really sick and needed to go home and which kids just weren't quite ready for that spelling test. No matter the ailment, Mollie made every child who came in to see her feel special.

During one month, we got more calls from Mollie than we had the whole previous year. The first one was that Alex wasn't feeling great. He had a headache and fever, and she thought my wife, Jeanne, should come and get him. Jeanne took him to the doctor's and sure enough, he had strep throat. He went on antibiotics and returned to school. Within a couple of weeks, he was back in Mollie's office with the same symptoms. Jeanne got the call and whisked him back to be seen by our pediatrician. Again, his strep test was positive, so he went on another antibiotic and was soon better. When my wife got her third call from Mollie in as many months, she said in exasperation, "He can't have strep throat again. It's just not possible!" But sure enough he did. We even had him tested to see if he was a carrier, someone who just had the bacteria living harmlessly in his throat, but the test came back negative. Frustrated, Jeanne called me and said, "Here you are a doctor and we keep sending our kid to school sick. I thought you couldn't get the same infection twice. What's going on?" While it didn't make Jeanne feel like a much better parent, it was reassuring to learn that with an infection like strep, there are enough different disease-causing bacterial strains for you to get it over and over again. The immunity you get from your first infection doesn't protect you against all the other strains.

Your immune system is remarkable. Among its many functions, it is an extremely sophisticated defense, constantly on guard for a wide array of common microbial invaders. In some cases, your immune system is strong enough to eliminate potentially dangerous ones the first time they even attempt to infect your body. In other cases they infect you but the immune system "remembers" how to fight the invader, making it unlikely that you will experience that infection again.

The idea that you cannot be infected by the same pathogen more than once likely stems from this concept of immunity—one dependent upon the "memory" of past invaders that your body's defense system largely keeps in immune cells known as memory B cells. If a familiar invader infects the body, these cells can quickly sound the alarm, activate your disease-fighting systems, and generate specific antibodies needed to fight off the infection.

This immune memory can be generated in different ways: It can develop after a naturally occurring infection or following a vaccination. The art of designing an effective vaccine is to create one that stimulates an immune response in your body that will last your lifetime without causing the illness you are trying to prevent. This isn't so easy to do. The protection you receive from many vaccines is lifelong; for other vaccines it fades over time.

With certain diseases, once you have them, you are done. For example, it is highly unlikely that you will be infected with the exact same strain of flu twice; people did not come down with smallpox more than once; and when you have had measles you can cross it off the list. Unfortunately, the microbial world is pretty smart and finds ways to evade your immune system; small changes to some microbes allow them to bypass your immune system and cause infection again. For example, flu viruses continually mutate and change, leaving you at renewed risk for infection from new strains. That is why you need an annual flu shot. For other infections, your immunity begins to fade over time, leaving you vulnerable to infections against which you were once protected. That is why you need booster shots for diseases like tetanus and whooping cough. There are also medical conditions and medications that can interfere with your ability to mount a strong immune response.

For all these reasons, when it comes to infectious diseases, the best defense is to never let your guard down. Make sure you are fully vaccinated (including being up to date with your boosters) and practice good hand-washing. Even if you've had "it" before, watch out. Never say you never have to worry.

DR. B'S BOTTOM LINE:

While your immune system is very good at recognizing many invaders and preventing disease the second time you are infected, it is not fail-safe. It is important to remember, though, that for many diseases it is not only possible to be sick only once, it is possible to never get sick from them at all—thanks to vaccines!

50

IS REST THE BEST THING FOR BACK PAIN?

Back pain is one thing I know about all too well. I've had back issues since I was a teenager. It's one of the downsides of being six foot six and walking upright; it puts a lot of strain on my lower back. All through my twenties, a couple of times a year my back would "go out." A strange term, but for me it meant excruciating pain traveling down my legs to my feet. It might come on while playing sports or just by simply getting out of bed. When this would happen, I would be incapacitated. Twice in my thirties, I blew a disc and needed operations to take the pressure off my nerve roots. Not fun.

I am not alone when it comes to knowing back pain. According to the NIH, nearly everybody has some that interferes with his or her day-to-day activities. It is one of the most common health-related reasons employees take off work and is the leading cause of job-related disability.

The back is a pretty complex structure composed of bones, muscles, ligaments, tendons, nerves, and discs all living together in very tight quarters. When everything works well, it is truly a thing of beauty. However, with aging, little changes start to happen. Back pain begins for most of us between ages thirty and fifty. As we age, bone strength and muscle elasticity and tone begin to decrease. The discs, which provide cushioning between your vertebrae, begin to lose fluid and flexibility, like old shock absorbers in a car. The passages between the vertebrae that allow nerves to pass can get constricted, causing pressure on the nerve roots and pain.

Many times pain begins after an injury or trauma from an accident: Lifting something too heavy, sudden movement, overexertion, or even overstretching. My worst episode of back pain came from doing exactly what I wasn't supposed to do: Lifting with my back instead of my legs. I was leaning over into the trunk of my VW Golf to lift out a very heavy television set. There was no way to lift it without taking the weight in my lower back. All of a sudden I went down; it felt like I had been shot in the back. Three days later I was in the operating room having the pressure from a blown disc relieved.

However, physical trauma isn't the only cause of back pain. When I'm stressed out, the tension tends to settle in my back. My shoulders tighten, my lower back goes into spasm, and I know I'm in for trouble. Obesity, poor physical condition, bad posture, smoking, pregnancy, stress, and sleeping "funny" can contribute to low back pain. Back pain can also result from arthritis or degenerative conditions in the bones or discs.

It used to be that when my back began to act up I'd head for bed to lie down until it felt better. It made intuitive sense. If you twist your ankle, you rest it until it is less tender, so why not your back? Well, it turns out that rest is not best when it comes to your back. While one to two days of rest shouldn't be harmful, a 1996 Finnish study was one of the first to find that people who continued their regular activities without bed rest appeared to have better back flexibility than those who rested in bed for a week. Other studies suggest that bed rest alone may actually make back pain worse and can lead to secondary complications including depression, decreased muscle tone, and blood clots in your legs.

If back pain strikes you, talk to your doctor to determine the most effective combination of prescription drugs and over-the-counter analgesics to reduce inflammation and discomfort. For most people, lower back pain goes away within a few days when treated with a combination of pain relievers, moderate activity, and gentle exercise. Let your doctor know if you are currently taking any other medications before they prescribe new ones. Although cold and hot compresses have never been scientifically proven to quickly resolve low back injury, I find them helpful. Try them and see. You can apply the cold compress to the injured area several times a day for up to twenty minutes for two to three days. After that, apply heat for brief periods to relax muscles and increase blood flow. Warm baths may also help relax muscles. Gentle exercises that help keep muscles moving can speed recovery by strengthening your back and abdominal muscles. Any mild discomfort felt at the start of gentle exercising should disappear as muscles become stronger. If your pain persists and lasts more than fifteen minutes, you should stop exercising and contact a doctor. Most back pain should improve with these treatments, although some discomfort might linger.

DR. B'S BOTTOM LINE:

If you have back pain, try to keep active with moderate activity, gentle exercise, and anti-inflammatory drugs. If you don't feel better after three days or if you have any muscle weakness or sensory changes, call your doctor.

TIPS FOR PREVENTING BACK PAIN

- Maintain a healthy diet and weight. Added fat, especially around your middle, puts a lot of pressure on your back.
- Remain active; incorporate exercise that maintains core strength, such as yoga or Pilates. Abdominal strength helps support your back muscles. Warm up gently before exercising or engaging in other physical activities.
- Try to reduce stress through yoga, meditation, and massage. Yoga can also help you improve your posture, flexibility, and balance.
- Don't hunch over. Proper posture will protect your back from injury. While standing, place both feet on the floor, with your shoulders back and weight distributed evenly over both legs. While sitting, make sure your desk and chair are sized properly for you. Hips and knees should be at ninety-degree angles, with your wrists and head in a neutral position. Use a chair that gives you good lumbar support or use an insert if your seat doesn't provide comfort. This applies to your car seat as well.

- Lift with your knees, keeping the object close to your body. Ask for help if you need to lift something heavy.
- Watch how heavy your backpack, briefcase, or purse is.
- Don't smoke; it impairs blood flow to spinal tissues.

51

IF NO ONE IN MY FAMILY HAS HAD BREAST CANCER, CAN I STILL GET IT?

I'll never forget the phone call my wife got fourteen years ago. She had just called her best friend, Sarah, to tell her she was pregnant with our second child. Sarah had some news to share as well: She had just been diagnosed with breast cancer. She was thirty-nine, a mother of two kids under ten, and had no family history of breast cancer. My wife and she were dumbfounded—how could this happen? What they didn't realize is that most women who get breast cancer *don't* have a relative who had it.

Ever since researchers discovered mutations in two important breast cancer susceptibility genes, BRCA1 and BRCA2, the genetic component linking relatives with their likelihood of developing the disease has gotten a lot of attention. If you inherit certain mutations in these genes, you have an increased risk for developing breast cancer, particularly at a young age. Considering the publicity that these genes have gotten, and the link with family history, one could be forgiven for thinking that they are responsible for most breast cancer cases. Here's what may surprise you: A look at the statistics proves this to be a misconception. Only 5 to 10 percent of breast cancer cases are considered to be hereditary (caused by a BRCA mutation or another known genetic link). Another 10 to 15 percent are classified as being familial (breast cancer runs in your family but no gene has been found yet to explain the risk). This means that 75 to 85 percent of breast cancers are likely to be nonhereditary in nature, just as in Sarah's case.

While women who inherit the BRCA genes may have up to an 80 percent chance of developing breast cancer, the important thing to remember is that women without this mutation, the *majority* of women, have a risk over their entire lifetime of closer to 12 percent. Most cases of breast cancer occur in that low-risk group because far more women do not have the BRCA mutation than have it.

Another misconception that surrounds the disease is that many people incorrectly equate a diagnosis of breast cancer as a death sentence. Not only is breast cancer *not* the leading cause of death for women, it isn't even the leading cancer killer. While breast cancer is far and away the most common type of non-skin cancer in women, when you look at cancer deaths, the picture is markedly different. Overall, for those who get breast cancer, the five-year survival rate is 89 percent, quite high when compared to many other cancers. Twice as many women die from lung cancer each year as die from breast cancer. Given that 80 percent of lung cancer is linked to smoking and is therefore preventable, why isn't more being done to focus on eliminating that risk?

Most likely it's because breast cancer resonates with women on many levels. Unlike the more equal-opportunity cancers, it rarely targets men. It also triggers body image issues associated with treatment, and, given its prevalence, has personally touched the lives of most women—forming an emotional connection to the disease. Additionally, awareness groups are experts at keeping the disease at the top of our minds. Hardly a month goes by when I don't sponsor a friend or colleague doing a walk or run to raise money for breast cancer research. I can't see the color pink without thinking about the disease. But there is a potential downside: It diverts attention from other conditions that could have a more significant impact on women's health. For example, the leading cause of death for women is the same as for men: Heart disease. A survey conducted by the American Heart Association in 2005 found that only 55 percent of women knew this. This lack of knowledge really matters. Women who realized that heart disease was the leading killer were more likely to take steps to lower their risk.

So make sure you work to prevent breast cancer, but don't forget that taking care of your health doesn't stop there.

DR. B'S BOTTOM LINE:

Family history is a crucial consideration when it comes to many cancers, including breast cancer. However, it is only one piece of the puzzle. Most women who have had breast cancer did not have a family history. There are a number of other factors that explain the bulk of breast cancer cases, and many factors that we don't yet know of. Remember that you do have control over some aspects of risk in the lifestyle choices you make.

GOOD CHOICES, REDUCED RISK

Given that the vast majority of breast cancers do not occur in those women with a known genetic marker or a strong family history, all women need to be aware of their modifiable risk factors and take action to reduce them.

- Maintain a healthy weight. The American Cancer Society warns of the link between being overweight and increased cancer risks, especially in postmenopausal women. Being overweight can cause your body to produce and circulate more estrogen and insulin, hormones that can stimulate cancer growth. It suggests keeping your body mass index below 25.
- Watch your alcohol consumption. Several studies have shown a link between alcohol consumption and elevated breast cancer risk, even at low levels of consumption. If you have a family history of breast cancer you might want to cut out alcohol. For others, you have to weigh the possible heart-related benefits of an occasional drink against the small increase in breast cancer risk that may result.
- Stop smoking. Do you need another reason to quit? Here's one! While the data aren't ironclad, there may be a link especially for women who

start young and are heavy smokers. Call 800-QUIT-NOW (800-784-8669) for help.

• Exercise. The risk of breast cancer, among other cancers, appears to be higher among couch potatoes. Keeping physically active not only helps improve weight and fitness, but it may also cut breast cancer risk.

• Get screened regularly. Mammograms are recommended every two years for all women fifty to seventy-four years old. For women younger than fifty, discuss risks and benefits of screening with your doctor to decide if you want earlier screening.

52

ARE HEART ATTACK SYMPTOMS THE SAME IN MEN AND WOMEN?

I don't wish a heart attack on anyone, but particularly, I don't wish one on a woman. It isn't because I'm gallant (although I like to think I am); it's because a heart attack in a woman is more likely to be missed, misdiagnosed, and undertreated. And when it comes to heart attacks, time is everything.

Here's why. During a heart attack, blood flow to some of the heart muscle is reduced or cut off, usually by a plaque or a clot in an artery. When this happens some heart muscle dies. If a significant amount dies, the heart may stop pumping entirely and the patient could die. Treatment is directed at restoring blood flow as quickly as possible to minimize the amount of muscle damage and improve heart function and chances of survival. This can be done by administering a clot-busting drug or by inserting a thin tube into the blocked artery to open it up.

Although heart disease is sometimes thought of as a "man's disease," it is actually an equal-opportunity killer. As the leading cause of death in both men and women in the United States, it is responsible for one in every four deaths among women. And, despite the larger role breast cancer detection plays in our conversation about women's preventative health, a woman is seven and a half times more likely to die from heart disease than from breast cancer.

When you think of the symptoms of a heart attack, what comes to mind? Here are some that might: Crushing chest pain that may shoot down an arm, heart palpitations, shortness of breath, and sweating. These iconic descriptions are typical male symptoms that have been well publicized. While chest pain is still the leading symptom in women, it is not unusual to see a different set of subtler symptoms. Women are more likely than men to report unusual fatigue, indigestion, sleep disturbance, and shortness of breath. The pain they feel may be just in the neck, back, or jaw.

Not only are women slower to identify their symptoms as those of a heart attack; they are also more likely to delay treatment. They often discount their ailments, thinking they are stress-related or gastrointestinal, and are reluctant to call 911. All of these delays can have serious consequences. And it gets worse. Once a woman gets to the hospital she is likely to get less treatment for her heart attack than a man. It takes a strong advocate to make sure that the right diagnosis is made and that treatment starts promptly.

DR. B'S BOTTOM LINE:

Women need to be aware that their heart attack symptoms may be very different from men's. Whether you have classic symptoms, such as chest pains, or more ambiguous symptoms of fatigue and indigestion, know the signs. *Everyone,* if you think you might be having a heart attack, call 911 and say, "I think I am having a heart attack." Then crush up an aspirin and swallow it (it can prevent further clot formation), sit down, and wait for the ambulance to come. Get to the hospital and demand a thorough evaluation. It's okay to be wrong, but if you are right, you might just have saved your own life.

RISKY BUSINESS

Know which heart disease risk factors you can't change and those you can. Anything you can do adds up over time and could save your life.

RISK FACTORS YOU CAN'T NECESSARILY CHANGE, BUT NEED TO BE AWARE OF:

- Family history of heart disease: Did your father or brother have a heart attack before age fifty-five? Did your mother or sister have one before age sixty-five? If so, you are more disposed to heart disease.

- Age: Are you over age fifty-five? Or, if you are a woman, are you younger but postmenopausal? Women are more likely to get heart disease once they have a drop in estrogen production. Other risk factors also tend to increase in middle age.

RISK FACTORS YOU CAN CHANGE:

- If you smoke, stop.
- If you have high cholesterol, diabetes, or high blood pressure, take efforts to control them.
- If you are overweight or obese, lose weight.
- If you are inactive, start exercising.

53

CAN I CALL IN SICK WITH A COLD?

Every year my children's elementary school would end with an awards ceremony. One of the honors was for perfect attendance. Through the roar of the applause for these kids, my wife and I would turn to each other and simultaneously mouth the words "Typhoid Marys." While we understood the school wanted to recognize these kids for their efforts to get to school (not to mention that the school was reimbursed for every day a student was there), we were convinced the determination to attend came more from parents who wanted to get them to school. We were also fairly certain that one of these kids was the child sneezing all over my son, causing my wife to have to take the day, or week, off from work to care for him after he came down with a terrible cold.

Our conditioning to get somewhere even when we feel terrible carries over even as we age. You know the feeling. You wake up in the morning with a sore throat, a headache, and a stuffy nose. You know you're sick and the only question that remains is whether you will spend the rest of the day on the couch or "tough it out" and head into the office.

Had you woken up with the high fever, body aches, and weakness typical of a bout of the flu, it's unlikely you would be having this internal debate; you probably would have had no choice but to stay in bed. But when it comes to the common cold, we tend to judge ourselves to be simply "under the weather" and show up to work despite our symptoms—often to the chagrin of our coworkers, who can't help but notice the crumpled tissues littered around our desks.

It turns out they have reason to be dismayed. The phenomenon known as "presenteeism" is widely recognized among infectious disease experts to be a problem. One of the factors that contributes to presenteeism seems to be a general misunderstanding of exactly *how* sick is *too* sick to show up for work. There is a feeling that you are doing people a favor by coming in. Not only do people who come to work despite feeling unwell tend to be less productive; they also expose their coworkers to their illness, further threatening health and productivity within the workplace.

Another contributor to presenteeism is a workplace that does not have a liberal sick leave policy and an economy in which staying home increasingly means not getting paid. This was a big issue in 2009 during the pandemic of influenza. When I was the acting director of the CDC, one of the key public health messages we put forward was for people to stay home when they were sick. In theory this made a lot of sense: Limit the contact people had with others when they are sick and you will reduce the spread of disease in the community. However, we lack a safety net in America to allow large numbers of people to stay home when ill. A survey conducted by Robert Blendon and colleagues at the Harvard School of Public Health found that if parents needed to stay home for seven to ten days to take care of themselves or a sick child, 44 percent thought that they might lose pay and have money problems and 25 percent reported that they were likely to lose their job. According to the Bureau of Labor Statistics, forty million private sector employees have no paid sick leave. It makes it hard to do what is best.

So given that it is frequently too difficult to do the right thing, when should you stay home? Here are four questions to consider:

- Are you contagious and is your illness dangerous? The common cold is contagious, but it tends to be more annoying than dangerous unless it is spread to someone with an immune disorder. It also spreads to others before you have symptoms (though you spread it more once you are coughing and sneezing).
- Are you well enough to do your job? If you aren't, there really isn't much value in going to work.
- Do you work in a setting where you can reduce your contact with others and limit spread? If you have a door you can close, you're in good shape. If you are dealing face-to-face with coworkers or customers all day, you're putting others at risk. In our newsroom, the senior producers work around a large table with less than a foot between workstations. Our *World News* anchor, Diane Sawyer, is quick to send home

anyone who comes in sick. She knows that is the only way to keep the whole team healthy.

• Would you like your colleagues to stay home if they were as sick as you are? Make sure you don't hold yourself to a higher standard than you would others.

Your answers to those questions should help you decide what to do.

If your work supports you taking the day off (and it should!), clear off the couch, break out the orange juice, and find your favorite daytime drama, preferably on ABC! You can catch up on lost time at work when you are feeling better in a couple of days.

DR. B'S BOTTOM LINE:

Calling in sick to the office is pretty easy when your symptoms are severe. If you are still able to walk around despite your symptoms, as is often the case with the common cold, this may seem like a harder call to make. The important thing to keep in mind when you are sick is that you are often doing your office mates, as well as your employer, a big favor by staying home. While your absence for a day or so may mean lost productivity, infecting others multiplies the problem.

SHOULD I CALL IN SICK?

STAY HOME:

These illnesses are very contagious and can be easily spread:

• The flu: Stay home until your fever has been gone at least twenty-four hours.

- Stomach bug: If you have a fever, see blood in your bowel movement, or become dehydrated, call a doctor.
- Strep throat: Stay home for twenty-four hours after the start of antibiotics.

GO TO WORK:

If you are up to it, these illnesses are not contagious:

- Allergies
- Sinus infection
- Back pain
- Hangover
- Headache
- Poison ivy
- Earache

YOUR CALL:

If you can contain the spread of illness by good handwashing and isolation and want to go to work:

- Cold
- Pinkeye

54

CAN I DIE OF A BROKEN HEART?

We've all heard the adage that someone died of a broken heart. While the concept sounds romantic, it is anything but. When a loved one dies, the pain is so palpable. While for most of us it's only an emotional trauma, it turns out that there is an actual medical condition based on physical symptoms, called broken heart syndrome. It is the name for sudden heart failure following a major shock, like the death of someone close to you.

Japanese doctors first recognized this syndrome in the early 1990s. They thought the enlarged heart that characterizes this condition, when seen on X-rays, looked like the flowerpot-shaped Japanese octopus trap, *takotsubo,* and named it as such. Also known as stress cardiomyopathy, it almost exclusively affects postmenopausal women.

It may be that as many as 1 to 2 percent of patients who are diagnosed with a heart attack in the United States are actually suffering from broken heart syndrome. While the symptoms are similar to heart attacks and can include chest pain, shortness of breath, and an irregular heartbeat, what is actually happening to your heart is totally different. A heart attack occurs when the muscle doesn't get enough oxygen to meet its needs, usually due to a blocked artery. It leads to permanent heart muscle damage. Broken heart syndrome may present in the same way, but there is no blockage in blood flow. It is likely the result of a surge in adrenaline and other hormones that overwhelm the heart muscle and inhibit its ability to pump properly. The heart takes on a different appearance. The left ventricle becomes swollen, but the rest of the heart functions normally.

Broken heart syndrome can be caused by both emotional and physical stress. Many of the women who suffer from it are healthy and active, not people you'd expect to have a heart problem. Stressors can come in all shapes and sizes, some related to sadness and some more generally connected to higher states of agitation. In a report in the *New England Journal of Medicine,* doctors from Johns Hopkins University documented cases as a result of deaths in the family, heated arguments, public speaking—even a surprise birthday party! Experts aren't sure why middle-aged women are at greater risk for a broken heart, but differences in hormones are one possible cause.

While broken heart syndrome can be fatal, almost all patients recover fully without any residual heart damage. It recurs in a small percentage of women and unfortunately there doesn't seem to be any way to prevent it.

DR. B'S BOTTOM LINE:

In stressful situations, if you feel like you are experiencing heart-attack-like symptoms, seek treatment right away, but don't assume it's a heart attack. Let your doctor know if you have just experienced an unusually emotional event. While very rare, you can die of a "broken heart."

55

DO CELL PHONES CAUSE BRAIN CANCER?

When you enter the hardware store near my home, you pass a sign requesting that you turn off your cell phone. When I questioned why the store was a "quiet zone," the owner replied it had nothing to do with noise reduction. He had brain cancer and didn't want to risk that radiation released by cell phones in the store could worsen it. I'm sure there's nothing anyone could say about the absence of solid proof that cell phones cause brain cancer that would change his mind.

About 227 million Americans own a cell phone and most use it every day (some people it seems are on it every minute). What really happens to you when you hold a small, electromagnetic-wave-emitting device against your ear for hours on end? Do the waves penetrate your skull? Do they have any effect on your brain?

For years the scientific community has been trying to address these questions, searching for evidence of any danger. They have examined the issues from every angle: Exploring the effects of radiation on the brain, tracking brain cancer rates over the years of increased cell phone use, and comparing brain cancer patients' cell phone usage to those without cancer. Thus far, the overwhelming majority of studies have not supported any connection between cell phone usage and damaging effects, let alone cancer, but that has done little to quell worries among the public. Let's examine the research.

While we know that cell phones emit radiation, not all radiation causes cancer. For our purposes, you can divide radiation into two groups: Ionizing and non-ionizing. Ionizing radiation is produced by X-rays and UV light and has the ability to directly damage DNA in your cells. By doing so, it can cause cancer. Cell phones emit an entirely different kind of radiation. They work by using electromagnetic energy, a form of non-ionizing radiation that produces radiofrequency (RF) waves, similar to FM radio waves and microwaves. Those RF waves go from your phone to the cell tower transmitting your signal. While RF waves don't damage DNA directly, at high levels RF waves can produce heat that can penetrate tissues. One small study looked at what happened to your brain when you held a cell phone up to your head for fifty minutes. It found a 7 percent increase in how your brain uses glucose in the area nearest the phone antenna. However, the study's authors make an important point: It isn't known whether the increased brain glucose metabolism is good, bad, or irrelevant.

From an epidemiological standpoint, if cell phone use causes brain cancer, we should have seen a similar upsurge in the disease as cell phones became more popular. The National Cancer Institute, which tracks cancer rates in the United States, found no increase in the rate of brain cancers between 1987 and 2007, the period of rapid increase in the use of cell phones. Data from Scandinavia, a region that was one of the first to introduce cell phones, similarly has found no increase in brain cancers. However, given that some cancers develop slowly, epidemiologists will continue to monitor these trends.

Many researchers have also looked at who developed brain cancer to determine if their cell phone usage was different from that of people who did not develop brain cancer, but the results have been inconclusive. In 2000, the international scientific community attempted a definitive study called Interphone. It was the largest study ever undertaken of cell phone use and brain cancer and included more than five thousand people with brain cancer, in thirteen different countries, all of whom were matched to similar people who did not have cancer. Unfortunately, the results actually caused more confusion than clarity. For those people who used cell phones the most, they did find an *increased* risk for two types of brain tumors, gliomas and meningiomas, especially on the side of the head that was their usual side for using their cell phone. But they found that people who used cell phones regularly had *lower* rates of brain cancer than people who never used cell phones. In fact, for everyone except those in the highest group of users, cell phone use *decreased* the risk of brain cancer. This does not make sense biologically. Normally there would be some adverse effect in occasional and moderate users if high users were developing cancer. Instead it showed beneficial outcomes of using cell phones. The conflicting results within the same study were attributed to bias and problems with the study itself. So much for clarity!

Worries were stoked recently when the WHO's International Agency for Research on Cancer added cell phones to a long list of exposures that are possibly carcinogenic in humans. Their approach is to include any item with a *possible* cancer link, to encourage future research and to alert those who are risk-averse to change their behavior. To be on this list, which includes everything from gasoline to pickled vegetables, there only has to be minimal evidence of a connection.

So where does that leave us today? The scientific evidence thus far does not support a connection between cell phone use and cancer. It doesn't make sense biologically and I am somewhat reassured by the stable brain cancer rates. However, I understand the concerns. This is a constantly changing arena and there is uncertainty given so many conflicting studies. But unlike environmental risks, over which you have little control, the use of cell phones is totally optional. If you are worried about developing cancer from using a cell phone, don't use one! There are still many people who only use conventional phones. If you need to use a cell phone and are concerned, then minimize your exposure by using a hands-free device, such as Bluetooth or the speakerphone function. Texting instead of talking will also reduce your exposure by increasing the distance from the phone to your head. If you must speak on the phone, keep your calls short.

One last thing. I can't leave this topic without a bit of a rant. While there is some debate about dangers of cell phone use and cancer, there should be *no* debate that cell phones can be dangerous. Cell phones in the car are a clear menace and there should be more uproar about these risks. A study by researchers at the University of Utah found that a driver using a cell phone, handheld or hands-free, is as impaired as a person driving with a blood-alcohol content of .08 percent (above the legal limit in most states). Texting while driving is even worse. It increases your risk of having an accident almost twenty-five-fold. If you are really concerned about cell phones and health, here is where your focus should be.

DR. B'S BOTTOM LINE:

There has been no plausible explanation for exactly how the low-level, non-ionizing radiation emitted by a cell phone could cause brain tumors. Given the dramatic increase in worldwide cell phone use, the fact that there has been no corresponding surge in the cases of brain cancer weakens the chances of a true relationship. However, it's easy to make simple changes to reduce your exposure. If you are really concerned about cell phones and your health, whatever else you decide to do, add this to the list: Turn yours off the next time you get in your car.

CELL PHONES AND KIDS

There is much less experience with cell phone exposure in the young. Our children are the first generation to grow up with very early and frequent exposure to cell phones. Although it isn't clear to me how cell phones could cause cancer, if there were a small risk to their developing brains it might not have shown up yet in cancer statistics. Cell phone technology is also changing. For now, if you are concerned, set limits on how the phone can be used. Have your kids use cell phones for texting and emergency calls and use landlines for longer conversations. Better yet, encourage them to have face-to-face conversations. Wouldn't that be a nice change?

56

WHAT SHOULD I DO IF I THINK I'M HAVING A STROKE?

In 2010, Beau Biden, the forty-one-year-old Delaware attorney general and son of Vice President Joe Biden, had a stroke. That's right, a stroke suffered by someone in his forties. While the risk for stroke goes up as you age, 10 to 15 percent of strokes occur in people younger than forty-five, making it critical for everyone to know the signs and symptoms to help themselves and others.

Here are some: Numbness and weakness on one side of the body. Confusion. Slurred speech. By any measure, these should be alarming symptoms. Yet in many cases, those who experience these telltale signs of stroke ignore them. According to the National Stroke Association, 42 percent of adult stroke sufferers wait an average of thirteen hours, and up to twenty-four hours, after the onset of symptoms before heading to the hospital.

Stroke is currently one of the leading causes of death and disability. On average, every forty seconds someone in the United States has one, which adds up to almost eight hundred thousand strokes per year. Strokes that are not deadly can lead to paralysis, permanent speech impairment, and emotional problems.

There are two basic types of strokes: Ischemic strokes, in which blood flow to part of the brain is cut off, and hemorrhagic strokes, in which a blood vessel in the brain bursts. Ischemic strokes are nine times more common than hemorrhagic ones, but both damage brain tissue.

Individuals who are at an increased risk of having a stroke include smokers, those with high blood pressure, heart disease, or diabetes. Individuals who have had transient ischemic attacks (TIAs)—"mini" strokes— are also at risk. TIAs occur when there is temporary blockage in an artery that keeps the brain from getting the blood it needs. Symptoms can last for just a few minutes or hours and can be warning signs that a bigger episode could be coming.

In nearly any case of stroke, early treatment is linked to a higher chance of surviving with the least amount of permanent neurological damage. This is especially true for ischemic strokes. With this type of stroke, administration of a clot-busting chemical known as tissue plasminogen activator, or tPa, has been shown to limit damage if it is given early enough after the onset of symptoms. This approach was confirmed in a 1995 study published in the *New England Journal of Medicine* that looked at hundreds of stroke patients and found that those treated within three hours after symptoms first appeared had a greater chance of being alive three months after their ordeal. If you wait too long to go to the hospital, you risk damage to more brain tissue and may miss the time frame during which tPa can work.

Yet, considering that most stroke victims wait at least thirteen hours before seeking care, it is clear that most Americans experiencing a stroke are missing this narrow window of benefit. Even patients who know the warning signs of a stroke—those who have had a stroke before—were unlikely to seek care soon enough because they did not judge their symptoms as serious. This needs to change.

To encourage people to take action and avoid denial, the National Stroke Association has a quick set of tips for determining whether someone is experiencing a stroke, so quick action can be taken. Known by its acronym, FAST, it involves the following memorable pointers:

- FACE: Ask the person to smile. Does one side of the face droop?
- ARMS: Ask the person to raise both arms. Does one arm drift downward?
- SPEECH: Ask the person to repeat a simple phrase. Does it sound slurred or strange?
- TIME: If you observe any of these signs, call 911 immediately because time matters!

For this and more information, visit www.stroke.org/site/PageServer?pagename=SYMP.

DR. B'S BOTTOM LINE:

For stroke treatment, time is of the essence. The worst thing you can do when you are having the symptoms associated with a stroke is to ignore them or pretend that they are not serious. Don't make that mistake. If you or someone you know is exhibiting any of the signs of stroke, call 911 immediately.

TIPS FOR PREVENTING A STROKE

While early treatment is good, not having a stroke is even better. While these things are good for everyone to do, if you have had a stroke in the past, you are at risk of having another, especially if you don't focus on prevention.

- Control high blood pressure with diet, exercise, and medications.
- If you smoke, stop. Call the quit line to get help, 800-QUIT NOW (800-784-8669).
- Watch out for diabetes. Controlling your blood sugar reduces your risk.
- Keep your cholesterol in a normal range.
- Know your family history. Anyone in your family have a stroke?
- Don't ignore transient ischemic attacks. TIAs can have all of the symptoms of a stroke but the symptoms go away.
- If you drink, do so in moderation.
- Treat heart disease to prevent clots that can cause strokes from forming.

57

SHOULD I BE WORRIED IF I'M SHAPED LIKE AN APPLE?

My wife recently went for an eye examination and was shocked to find that her doctor had lost more than one hundred pounds from lap-band surgery. The doctor explained that although she knew she was overweight, what concerned her most was that she was holding it all in her middle. She knew that excess belly fat was a predictor for future health problems. My wife came home surprised that the optometrist's shape spurred her into action more than the numbers on the scale.

As if the list of things to watch for good health isn't long enough already, add body shape to the mix. Numerous studies have shown that where you put on your weight can have an effect on your health. No one likes to be referred to as a piece of fruit, but when it comes to body shapes that cause concern, it's as, well, comparing apples to pears.

Your particular body shape is determined partly by where you deposit fat. There are two types of fat: Subcutaneous and visceral. Subcutaneous fat is the under the skin, "pinch an inch" kind that most people commonly think of when they think of fat. Deposit your fat subcutaneously on your hips, thighs, and butt, and you will be more pear-shaped. Visceral fat is internal fat that is located around your organs. Deposit a lot of visceral fat in your belly and you will have a larger waist and appear more apple-shaped. Unlike subcutaneous fat cells, visceral fat cells are very metabolically active, producing hormones that can cause insulin resistance, a precursor to type 2 diabetes.

In some studies, the relationship of your waist measurement to your hip measurement is more closely tied to early, hidden signs of heart disease than other common measures of obesity, including your body mass index (BMI) and the waist circumference alone. Although the importance of body shape has not been accepted by the entire medical community, it hasn't stopped a veritable "belly fat" industry from pushing books, diets, and exercise regimens focused on reducing visceral fat.

Unfortunately, the reality is that a lot of what determines your shape is out of your control. If your parents were apples, you will have a predisposition toward becoming one, too. Women tend to put on more belly fat once they hit menopause; men put on more belly fat than women during their younger years. Although I am convinced by the science that belly fat is more dangerous than other fat, in the end I don't pay much attention to body shape. Here is why: It isn't that "pears" are at no risk and don't have to pay attention to their health. You can be pear-shaped and be quite unhealthy.

Regardless of which fruit you resemble, you need to do the same things to be healthy: Eat a balanced diet and get exercise. Aerobic exercise and an appropriate diet are great ways to reduce both visceral and subcutaneous fat, improve your cardiovascular health, and reduce your risk for diabetes and other diseases.

DR. B'S BOTTOM LINE:

Although the debate rages on, there does seem to be some validity to the idea that your waist size, and how it stacks up to your hip size, affects your risk for diabetes and heart disease. If you had your choice, you'd do better being born a pear than an apple. However, the fact is that carrying too much fat on your body is unhealthy, period. Instead of worrying about whether you are an apple or pear, aim to be the healthiest apple or pear you can be.

6

TAKE CONTROL OF YOUR HEALTH

*Your Questions on How to Avoid Getting Overtested,
Overtreated, and Harmed by Health Care*

It's scary being sick, especially if you have to question whether you are getting the best care possible. It's time to let you in on some of the secrets of medicine. You can take steps to make sure that when you have to interact with doctors and nurses and hospitals, you will have the best outcome. I've been practicing medicine for more than twenty-five years. During that time, I've seen some incredible physicians and nurses perform almost miraculous work, helping patients cope with enormous health burdens. I've trained physicians and seen the gift that some possess: How they are able to connect with their patients, understand their issues both physical and emotional, and empower their patients to make their health decisions. I've also seen some pretty horrendous doctors who lack the skills to practice the art of medicine. Doctors who leave their patients lost and confused.

The key to success when interacting with doctors is to realize that while your doctor is there for you, you are in charge and you have choices. So often in the relationship with health care, patients feel powerless and take what the doctor says as gospel. In this section, I'll share my advice as to how to make that relationship a truly positive one.

Regardless of the hand that fate might have dealt you, the most important thing you can do is to own your health. By that I mean, don't look to others to make the most personal decisions about your life. With many chronic diseases there may come a time when a specific course of treatment will present a complicated choice between longevity and quality of life. Who can make that decision for you better than you?

If you feel like more of an observer in your health and health care decision process, let's change that. Let's work on empowerment so that you feel like an active participant in partnership with your medical providers. By knowing yourself you can understand the risks arising from your own behaviors. By taking the time to explore your roots you can understand the risks that run in your family. This information will allow you to have a more open and honest relationship with your physicians and to understand the choices that you have to make.

First and foremost is who will be caring for you. Choosing your doctor should be based on many factors, the most important of which is whether you feel this is someone with whom you can share your most personal information. The best doctor for your friend might be the worst doctor for you. I'll help you figure out how to find the one who is right for you.

Medical protocols are constantly changing. Routine tests and exams you did without hesitation a year or two ago might not be in your best interest now. Before you agree to any test I'll help you sort out if it is right for you.

The truth is that you have the right to drive your own medical decisions based on your own assessments of risks and rewards. Your health belongs to you. No one can give it to you, nor should anyone be able to take it away.

58

DOES DOCTOR KNOW BEST?

When it comes to picking doctors who are right for you, I think the adage "Sometimes you have to kiss a lot of frogs to find your prince" rings true. We've all been in this situation: A doc is telling us what to do and we're nodding our heads but silently thinking, "Get me out of here!" I once went to a dentist who wanted to put crowns on all of my molars, just in case my old fillings gave out. I quickly made my exit and found one I was more in sync with. He declared my old metalwork, while not pretty, totally adequate. It's been almost twenty years since that first run-in and the fillings are still holding strong. Other times I didn't listen to myself, although I should have. There was the urologist I went to for my vasectomy. I thought because he was the chairman of the department, he'd be the best. He seemed a little disconnected, but I chalked that up to a lack of bedside manner. It turns out he was a lab scientist and hadn't done more than a few procedures in decades. When he stitched a little too much and I had to go back for a second surgery, I vowed in the future to ask more questions and be more prepared. Even for me, a physician, finding a good doctor has been difficult. I had to learn to take responsibility for my health so I could make better decisions.

A few years ago, when I took my job at ABC News, I moved from Atlanta to New Jersey, which meant I needed to find a new physician. I was determined to do better this time and asked a fellow doctor for a referral. He raved about one particular doctor, so I was feeling pretty confident when I went. I had no health complaints when I scheduled my first visit, but was turning fifty and knew I needed to get a referral for a colonoscopy. I filled out my paperwork and met him in his office to talk. He reviewed my forms, commented on my lack of medical problems, and then asked a few questions:

"Do you take a daily multivitamin?"

"No," I replied. "My wife loves to cook and we eat a very well-balanced diet. I get my nutrients through food."

"Well, I think you should take a multivitamin just in case," he said.

"Do you take a baby aspirin every day?" he then asked.

"No, I don't have risk factors for heart disease, and I am concerned that the risk of stomach bleeding outweighs the benefits for my heart," I answered.

"Well, I think all men should take a baby aspirin when they reach fifty."

"Okay," he went on. "Today we'll measure your PSA. Check you for prostate cancer."

"No thanks," I said. "The American Cancer Society recommends we talk about this. I've reviewed the evidence and for me, I don't think the benefits of a PSA outweigh the risks."

"I don't agree," he said. "If it's elevated, we can follow it. We don't need to do surgery automatically and besides, the surgeon I use is very good."

Whoa! We're talking about surgery when I didn't even want to take the blood test? I could tell at this point that we weren't a match. But I had already invested all this time. Should I just stick it out and do what he recommended? My friend thought so highly of this guy, after all. As tempting as it was to just hang in there, I said, "It seems like we have a different approach to health, and I think it would be better for me to see someone else." I made a few phone calls, asked some more questions, and found a doctor who had the same approach as I did: No supplements unless necessary and no procedures without sound medical justification. When she recommends something that I'm not sure about, we talk about it and she helps me make a choice that is right for *me*.

The bottom line is that a doctor-patient relationship should be about mutual trust and respect—about your doctor getting to know you and helping you make informed health decisions. Your doctors are your health consultants in this relationship, not the decision makers. The choices you make about your health are value-based. Only you know what is most important to you.

I recently was counseling a colleague whose father has incurable cancer. He was about to start chemotherapy. I asked her what her father hoped to accomplish with the treatment: Prolonging life or maximizing its quality. She wasn't sure and felt certain that the oncologist had not had that conversation with her dad. We talked about why that question was something only her father could answer. At times chemotherapy can help people live longer but at the cost of their quality of life, due to side effects from the drugs. This was a value-based decision as to what her father wanted, not a medical decision.

Remember, the basis of any good doctor-patient relationship is trust and open communication. It's all right to say no to something you don't want to do. It is important for you to be open with your doctor about your health, your risk tolerance, and any concerns you might have about what they are ordering or recommending. If they are not willing to have this talk with you or you don't feel comfortable having this conversation with them, it might be time to shop around for a new doctor

DR. B'S BOTTOM LINE:

When it comes to health, only you know what is best for you. Doctors may know more about what is physically going on with your body, and they may be able to provide information on the most likely outcomes of the choices that you make in terms of treatment. Ultimately, though, the choice is yours when deciding on treatment. The good doctor respects you and empowers you to own your own health.

59

HOW DO I STAY SAFE IN THE HOSPITAL?

Didn't it seem like there was a time when if you were really sick the hospital was the safest place to be? You knew there were doctors and nurses working around the clock to determine what ailed you. The only thing you needed to think about was getting well. Was that all a myth? Things seem a little different now. It's hard to miss the stories. Someone went into the hospital for something minor and never came home. Another went in for surgery on one leg and ended up being operated on the other. A friend of a friend went to the hospital for a minor procedure and ended up with an infection that almost killed him. No question—these are very scary stories. However, it's hard to tell whether these calamities are happening all the time or just getting a lot of attention due to the shock factor. Do you *really* have to worry about your health taking a turn for the worse when you are admitted to the hospital?

Unfortunately, you do. Hospitals can be very dangerous places and errors are stunningly common. A 2010 report from the inspector general in the U.S. Department of Health and Human Services found that 27 percent of people on Medicare who were hospitalized in 2008 were harmed while in the hospital, either seriously or temporarily. Almost half of these incidents were preventable. The reason we don't hear about these situations more often is equally concerning: Most never get reported.

A lot can go wrong:

- Medication errors: These come in many forms. You can get the wrong drug, too much of a drug, too little of a drug, a drug to which you have a known allergy, or a drug that interacts with some other drug you are on. The impacts depend on the drugs involved but can include bleeding, confusion, low blood sugar, and kidney failure.

- Surgical errors: A piece of surgical equipment like a sponge can be left in your body; you can have excessive bleeding during the operation; you can even have the operation performed on the wrong part of the body.
- Patient care errors: These include falling out of bed, getting a clot in your leg from not moving around enough, getting too much intravenous fluid, and bedsores.
- Infections: Whenever there is a tube entering your body or a break in the skin, you are at risk of getting an infection. These include infections from IVs, catheters, breathing tubes, and surgical sites. These infections are largely preventable.

Let's focus on the infections a bit more because the numbers here are staggering. Hospitals are full of sick people, many harboring very dangerous germs. According to the CDC, one in every twenty hospitalized patients will become infected with something while in the hospital. Not only are people getting infected; 16 percent are with germs that are super-resistant, many almost untreatable.

The death toll from these hospital-acquired infections in 2002 (the last year for which there are data) was nearly one hundred thousand! In many cases, the patients who are most affected are the ones who need to be in the hospital the most—patients in the intensive care unit.

So what's the solution? Clearly, if you need to go to the hospital for care, the risk of harm shouldn't keep you away. You can take some comfort that there are ongoing efforts to make hospitals safer, including programs to reduce surgical errors, medication errors, hospital-acquired infections, and falls. However, not all hospitals are the same; the more informed you are, the safer you will be. If you are going in for an elective procedure, go online and compare hospitals. Which hospital does more of them? Which has the lower complication rate? Both *Consumer Reports* and the Department of Health and Human Services have websites that provide some of this information, and you can find links to them in the Notes section at the end of this book. There are fewer mistakes made by doctors and hospitals with more experience. Ask your doctor where he or she would personally go to have the procedure done. It can be quite revealing.

Once you're there, these actions will help protect you in the hospital:

- Have an advocate with you. This is someone who knows you well and will pick up on any change in your behavior. They will speak for you when you can't. Are you acting confused? Do you have a new pain or fever? Your advocate will make sure the staff checks to see whether you have a new infection or a medication reaction. Pick someone who isn't afraid to speak up for you.

- Protect your body. Don't let anyone touch you whom you did not actually see wash her hands or use a hand sanitizer. It may be uncomfortable to ask, but you need to speak up and say, "Excuse me, did you wash your hands?" This will go far in reducing your chance of picking up an infection.

- Ask questions and don't be hesitant to speak up for yourself. If you have an IV or a urinary catheter in place, ask each day whether it is necessary and when it can come out. This will force your health care team to think about it. The longer that lines are in, the more likely they are to get infected.

I needed to draw on these resources recently. While on vacation, my dad was admitted to a small hospital because they thought he might be having a heart attack. Tests determined he had a blockage in his coronary arteries that would require having stents put in. I spoke to his doctor on the phone and found out that the hospital he was in did not have as much experience performing cardiac catheterizations as the one across town. I also learned that the hospital he was in did not have heart surgeons on site in case something went wrong and emergency surgery was needed. Not only that, but the hospital didn't have a relationship with the other nearby hospitals, so if there *was* a problem, they would have to airlift him to a hospital miles away! Based on this information, I moved my dad across town to the hospital that had more experience with this procedure and had the appropriate staff in case additional treatment was necessary. If I hadn't known to ask this, he would have been put at unnecessary risk.

While my dad was in the hospital, my mother or I was there at all times, making sure everyone who came into his room applied hand sanitizer. When I spoke with my dad's cardiologist I asked about the skill level of the specialist who would be performing the heart catheterization. I asked how many similar procedures this doctor had performed and what his complication rate was. I asked the cardiologist that if he himself needed this treatment done, would this doctor be his choice to perform it? Was it easy to ask all these questions? Absolutely not, even for me! In fact, one doctor was a bit taken aback. However, in the end my father got excellent care and he left the hospital in much better shape than when he went in. No errors, no infections. If we are all willing to ask the tough questions and advocate for ourselves and loved ones, doctors won't be surprised by these types of questions, and those horrifying stories will truly become the exceptions to the rule.

DR. B'S BOTTOM LINE:

It is unfortunate but true that being in the hospital when you are ill has risks besides what put you there. Don't put off care because you are worried about those added risks, but be aware of them. Appoint yourself (and your friends or family) as members of your health care team. Make sure you and a trusted person ensure you are getting the best care by knowing the right questions to ask—starting with the ones I asked for my dad—and more importantly, by not being too intimidated to ask them.

YOUR HOSPITAL CHECKLIST

When going to the hospital, make sure you:

- Provide the names of all the medications you are on, whether prescription or over-the-counter, to your doctor or nurse. Better yet, bring them with you so they can confirm dosages and other information. This includes everything, even vitamins and supplements. If you are taking any illegal or undocumented drugs, let them know that, too. If you are not forthcoming, it could affect your care.
- Inform the staff of any allergies you might have to both medications and food.
- Find out who is coordinating your care and ask for a game plan. Make sure you understand what is in store. Ask why you are having certain tests and when you should expect the results. A lot of anxiety can be avoided if you are prepared and know what's coming. If you are having surgery, ask details about the recovery process. I had a friend who had foot surgery and thought she would be back at work in a few days. It turned out that the typical recovery took more than two weeks.
- Read your discharge orders and go over them until you understand them. Know what medication to take and when to start taking it. Know what complications to look for or what would be considered out of the ordinary. Be clear about what to do if a problem arises, whether it requires a phone call, an office visit, or a trip to the ER.
- If you have a question or concern, don't be afraid to speak up! It's your body.

60

DOES WHERE A DOCTOR WENT TO MEDICAL SCHOOL MATTER?

My wife, Jeanne, and I had a whirlwind romance. When she told her best friend, Sarah, that she was moving across the country to be with me after dating for barely a month, Sarah asked how her parents took the news. Jeanne replied, "Are you kidding? An Ivy League doctor! What more could they want?"

For many parents, and patients, fancy medical school credentials carry a lot of weight. It's a safe bet that the first place many potential patients' eyes drift to when they enter a doctor's office is the back wall, specifically to the frame that holds that physician's medical degree. And it's easy to see why. Given how often we hear about the quality of institutions such as Harvard, Johns Hopkins, the University of Pennsylvania, and Stanford, one can be forgiven for automatically assuming that the doctors who hail from these top-rated schools naturally provide a better quality of care.

But is this really the case? Should you base your choice of physician on where they went to medical school? At the CDC I worked with brilliant doctors who trained at the most prestigious institutions in the country. Would I want many of them to be my or my family's caregivers? With their bedside manners, I don't think so. Most of them readily admit that they are just as unenthusiastic about the thought of seeing patients. They like being in the lab, in the field doing a study, or in the center of the public health policy world. As smart as they are, they never went into medicine intending to practice clinically.

Currently, the research examining the link between a doctor's medical school and the quality of care he or she offers is relatively sparse. However, there are some studies that suggest it matters little whether your doctor's shingle has an Ivy League name on it or not.

One of the best studies to look at this question was conducted by researchers at the University of Pittsburgh School of Medicine and the RAND Corporation. They looked at all the doctors practicing in Massachusetts and rated them in terms of quality on a wide range of measures. They then looked to see what characteristics were associated with providing higher quality of care. Surprisingly, the only factors that predicted quality of care at all were these: On a 100 percent scale, female physicians did better than male physicians by 1.6 percentage points, those with board certification did better than those without by around 3 percentage points, and American-trained physicians did better than internationally trained physicians by 1 percentage point. These differences were the only predictors that held up, and the impact of these factors was tiny! There was absolutely no relationship between quality of care and whether the doctor went to a medical school ranked in the top ten by *U.S. News & World Report*.

So if it isn't so important where they went to medical school, what should you know when it comes to choosing a primary care doctor? It's important to realize that there are many different types of doctors to choose from, each with his or her various strengths and advantages. No one doctor is right for everyone.

The first step is to understand what factors are important to you. Make a list. The National Library of Medicine offers a wealth of information and a number of tips to consider. These include logistical issues like office location, scheduling convenience, and type of insurance taken. Then there is style: Does the doctor order a lot of tests? Is her approach focused on maintaining and promoting health or on treating disease? I like a doctor who takes a very evidence-based approach to practice. My wife likes someone she feels comfortable talking to. My kids need someone with flexible hours who is willing to squeeze them in when the inevitable emergency occurs.

Then ask around. Friends and relatives might get you started. If you are moving, your current doctor might know some doctors elsewhere who have a similar style. If you have a particular medical condition, you can go to your disease's advocacy website to get some help with referrals or contact your health plan for doctors in your area.

Finally, set up an appointment to interview prospective doctors. As a pediatrician, I had expectant parents do this all the time. It gave them a chance to judge what I think is the most important factor in picking a doctor: Is this someone you can talk to? How are his communication skills? Is she a good listener? Will you be comfortable sharing some of your most personal concerns and information? Internists and family doctors may not agree to an informational appointment, but it doesn't hurt to ask.

Sometimes you go through all of this and still end up with a doctor who isn't right for you. It's okay to switch if it's not working. I did and now have a doctor who is wonderful! She and I can talk openly about my health, and I feel she really listens to my opinion about what I want to do, before she makes a recommendation.

In the end so much of the quality of care you receive will depend on the relationship you and your doctor develop. That determines whether your doctor is good or not—not the diploma hanging on the wall.

DR. B'S BOTTOM LINE:

Choosing a doctor is one of the most important health decisions you will make, so it pays to shop around. But judge the person, not the piece of parchment.

THE FIRST STEPS FOR CHOOSING A DOCTOR

Connecting with your doctor is the most important criterion in picking your physician, but don't ignore the little things. Check on their office hours, whether they take your insurance, and how responsive they are. If you call with a question, will your doctor call back or will it be a partner or nurse? How quickly can you expect a return phone call? How quickly can they squeeze you in if you are sick? How long is the wait time to schedule a physical? When you go for a visit, do they keep on time or are you in the waiting room for an hour? These are small things, but they have a big impact on the experience.

61

SHOULD I GET AN ANNUAL PHYSICAL?

How many times have you left your annual physical and said to the office staff, "See you next year"? For many, this visit, even when in good health, is a rarely neglected ritual. As much as you may be annoyed about the disruption in your schedule—not to mention donning those paper gowns—it is an age-old assumption that in order to stay well you must get a yearly check-up.

Surveys support that feeling. Most adults feel they should get an annual physical, and most doctors feel it is time well spent. We take our cars and our pets in for periodic service and examination, so why not ourselves? When we see the doctor, we want to be examined, head to toe, inside and out. We want to have "routine" tests performed: Blood pressure check, electrocardiogram, blood counts, and blood sugar measurement. And as uncomfortable as pap smears are, women expect to have one to look for cervical cancer. The same goes for men having their prostate glands palpated for any lumps or irregularities. It is reassuring to get that "clean bill of health" and know we are good to go for the year.

Unfortunately, there is very little evidence to show that you need to have these things performed every year or that doing so will lead to improved health in people who are feeling well. Annual pap smear? No longer recommended. Every three years is fine for most. Blood pressure check? Every two years will do. Prostate exam? Questionable value at all. Electrocardiogram? Not useful without heart symptoms or risk factors. Blood sugar measurement? The American Diabetes Association says to check it every three years unless you have high blood pressure or are obese, in which case you should check it more often. What about the actual exam? Shouldn't your doctor listen to your heart and lungs every year? Not really. There isn't much to support a physical examination unless you have symptoms of something that is bothering you. Many health professionals think a change to more selective screenings based on your personal and family history is warranted instead of a general "overhaul."

There are a number of preventive measures that have been shown to be beneficial and are recommended by the U.S. Preventive Services Task Force. However, these screening tests primarily have been shown to be valuable in specific populations based on risk. For example, I test all of my sexually active adolescent and young adult patients every visit for sexually transmitted diseases and HIV. For the most part they are at high risk for these diseases. If my patients were older individuals in long-term monogamous relationships, I wouldn't do this testing without symptoms. On the other hand, all patients should be asked about their use of tobacco products and, if they use them, whether they would like help in quitting. This is one screening test that can be beneficial.

Research has found that the people who get regular screenings are more likely to be at lower risk for disease than the general population but are still subjected to a battery of tests to check for a variety of diseases. The results of these tests have been shown to do little or nothing to discover, ward off, or prevent disease. Of course, there are times in our lives when routine visits are worthwhile: Regularly scheduled visits throughout childhood as you are developing emotionally and physically; throughout pregnancy; at certain milestone ages for cancer screening and cholesterol and blood pressure measurement. Unfortunately, the idea that many conditions are picked up on routine examination of an otherwise healthy person without risk factors before they become symptomatic, and that the earlier discovery makes a difference, is based on anecdotal evidence. It's just not the way it works. The vast majority of tests that are abnormal in people without symptoms are what are called false positive tests. They lead to more tests but they rarely lead to improved health.

In addition to unnecessary testing, here's the elephant in the room. Both doctors and insurance companies have to question the costs in time and dollars for long exams that don't lead to improved health. After all, these costs are passed on indirectly to consumers and business owners through higher premiums. Even if we might not pay out of pocket each time, we all contribute to general health care costs at work. More importantly, though, when you need to see a doctor for a sick visit, it probably won't make you feel better knowing you have to wait to get in because he's busy examining someone who's healthy and doesn't really need the visit.

So, if the research doesn't support the practice, is it possible that any good can come from seeing your doctor regularly, even when you are well? Definitely. I do think the visit can be valuable as long as most of it takes place sitting and talking with your clothes on. Sure, get your blood pressure checked (though you don't need to get that checked in your doctor's office; many times elevated blood pressure when you visit your doctor is what is called "white coat hypertension," an elevation just from the stress of being in your doctor's office); periodically check your cholesterol; and make sure your immunizations are up to date. But focus your time on your conversation with your doctor. That is when your doctor can look at your lifestyle and family history and help you identify behaviors that might lead to illness down the road. The periodic well visit should also be a way to develop the intangible benefits of a healthy and comfortable doctor-patient relationship that is useful if illness strikes.

To prepare for your visit, write down any questions since your last visit. Prepare a detailed family history so that you know what diseases you are most at risk for. Look at your lifestyle honestly: How much exercise are you getting? How much drinking do you do? How much sleep do you get? How is your diet? Open up to your doctor about your biggest health concerns and goals and see what advice you can get. That is when you get a sense as to whether your doctor and you really connect, which is so important when you are sick. The keys to good health lie in healthy behaviors, not in a lot of unnecessary invasive measures. Look to your doctor for advice on how to exercise more, eat better, stop smoking, and control your stress levels.

If 90 percent of your visit takes place in the examination room with you wearing one of those paper gowns, don't kid yourself into thinking that what you are doing is really good for your health. It's not.

DR. B'S BOTTOM LINE:

Most primary care physicians and patients agree that there is something good that comes out of the annual checkup. However, the weight of the evidence suggests that for healthy people the best thing that may result from these regular well visits is a closer doctor-patient relationship, not the early detection of disease. Ask which screening tests are appropriate for you and why. If you spend most of your time talking, your visit can be time well spent.

WHAT SCREENING TESTS DO YOU NEED?

Check these sources out. They will tell you what is recommended depending on your age and risk factors:

PREVENTIVE SERVICES RECOMMENDED BY THE U.S. PREVENTIVE SERVICES TASK FORCE
Agency for Healthcare Research and Quality,
www.ahrq.gov/clinic/pocketgd1011/gcp10s1.htm

MEN: STAYING HEALTHY AT ANY AGE
Agency for Healthcare Research and Quality,
www.ahrq.gov/ppip/healthymen.htm

WOMEN: STAYING HEALTHY AT ANY AGE
Agency for Healthcare Research and Quality,
www.ahrq.gov/ppip/healthywom.htm

62

SHOULD I ASK FOR A SECOND OPINION?

No one would dream of remodeling his house without interviewing several architects and getting multiple bids. Hearing what one says influences how you view another's ideas. You shop around to compare prices before making big purchases, for everything from a car to new kitchen appliances, to make sure you are getting the best price and the best service. My wife is the first to admit she wouldn't even dream of changing her hairstyle without polling friends to get their input. Every day you ask for second opinions and never think twice about it. It's a sign of being a knowledgeable consumer and making sure you've got the information you need to make informed decisions. Yet, when it comes to medical advice for serious conditions, many people are hesitant to get another point of view. And research shows that this reluctance may be bad for your health.

From a patient's perspective, medicine can come across looking pretty cut-and-dried. You see your doctor, tell your story, get examined, have tests done, and receive a diagnosis and treatment plan. You might assume that the result would be the same regardless of whom you see, who you are, and where you live. That couldn't be further from the truth. There are many nonclinical factors that affect your diagnosis, and there are glaring differences in treatment for the same condition by race, gender, region of the country, income, and health insurer. With all of those variables, why wouldn't everyone get a second opinion?

Routine second opinions have been shown to improve the diagnosis and treatment of a vast number of diseases, including breast cancer, colon cancer, liver cancer, thyroid cancer, prostate cancer, and lymphomas. They have even been shown to improve drug prescribing for attention deficit disorder. But most people don't ask for them.

A 2005 Gallup poll asked nearly five thousand Americans this question: "When your doctor diagnoses a condition, prescribes a treatment or operation, how often do you get a second opinion from another doctor?" Three percent said always, 41 percent said sometimes, and the most common response, at 49 percent, was never! There is an unfounded fear that challenging your doctor is disrespectful or insulting to him or her. A good doctor should welcome your inquiries and not be judgmental of your desire to get the most information possible. Many medical decisions come with consequences, and the risks and benefits should be explored and well documented.

Here are some of my top reasons for getting a second opinion:

- You will have more confidence in your doctor and less reservation about your course of action if you hear the same thing from more than one person. You will also have less regret if things don't all go according to plan.
- Some diagnoses are hard to make. If you have persistent symptoms despite your current therapy, see if someone else has something better to offer.
- Most conditions have alternative approaches to treatment and all treatment carries risk. Know what the options are so that you can make the best choice for you. You want to make sure that your style and your doctor's style match. If your doctor seems to be too aggressive or too laid-back for you, he or she probably is.
- Some doctors stay more current on cutting-edge treatments than others.
- Doctors see such a different mix of cases. For one doctor, you might be the only patient that month coming in with your ailment. For another doctor, you might be one of several that week.

Requesting a second opinion is hard to do! In my fantasy world your doctor would say to you, "Why don't I help you get another opinion on this? I'd love to hear what my colleagues have to say." Unfortunately, that doesn't happen very often, so here are two simple sentences that you can use if you ever have a serious illness or a critical medical decision to make. It's hardest to say the first time. After that it will come a bit more naturally.

"Doctor, that makes a lot of sense, but before we go forward with treatment, I'd like to get another opinion. Is there someone you'd recommend?"

DR. B'S BOTTOM LINE:

I know it isn't easy; challenging an authority figure rarely is. Good doctors should not take it as an insult or a challenge to their ability. In most cases, doctors will be more than willing to arrange for such a consultation, and they may even be happy that you asked. If you find that your doctor is resistant to this notion, it may not only be time for a second opinion—it may be time to get a new doctor.

ON SECOND THOUGHT

Before you visit a doctor for a second opinion, you should do the following:

- Ask your doctor for a recommendation of whom to see. Ask whom they would consult if they or a family member had the same ailment.
- Ask friends for recommendations.
- Check with your insurance provider to see if they cover second opinions. Many do. If yours doesn't, it still may be worth the investment, depending on the severity of the issue you are dealing with.
- Ask your doctor to send your medical records to the doctor giving the second opinion in time for your appointment. That way, the new physician can familiarize himself or herself with your needs and you may not have to repeat the tests you already had.
- Call the second doctor's office and make sure they have your records before you go.
- Write down a list of questions to take with you to the appointment.
- Don't go alone. It always helps to have someone with you, taking notes and helping to ask the tough questions.

63

IF MY DOCTORS ORDER A LOT OF TESTS, DOES THAT MEAN THEY'RE MORE THOROUGH?

I was talking to my mechanic recently and he confessed he hadn't had a physical in almost forty years. He had been treated for specific issues, and had seen doctors in that time, but when it came to an overall health exam, he said he was just too nervous to go. He confessed he was afraid of all the tests that are part of that type of visit. His brother had recently been misdiagnosed and had been put through a battery of tests, for naught.

Contrast this with the public outrage that went up when a government advisory body, the U.S. Preventive Services Task Force, recently changed the recommendations for screening tests for breast cancer, cervical cancer, and prostate cancer. They recommended less frequent testing for all three. "Outrageous," people said. "Clearly this is being driven by a concern for cost, not people's health. How dare they deny people these lifesaving tests!"

I don't think there is any issue that is harder for me to talk about on the air than the issue of overtesting. Most Americans like to be tested. They feel that routine screening tests are a great way to pick up problems before they become apparent and thereby prevent disease. I wish that were so. For many conditions testing is just not very good at distinguishing between abnormal results that indicate a problem and those that don't. It may be counterintuitive, but the results of a test for a person who has undergone testing because of specific symptoms have a much different meaning than those of someone who is healthy and is just getting a routine screening. For many diseases, unfortunately, earlier detection before symptoms develop doesn't make a difference.

Let's look at the chest X-ray. A routine chest X-ray was once part of the annual physical and the pre-employment examination, as well as a way of looking for lung cancer. A study published in 2011 in the *Journal of the American Medical Association* looked at whether routine chest X-rays improved survival from lung cancer. Clearly, if earlier detection made a difference, picking up lung cancer that way would lead to improved survival over picking it up once someone was symptomatic. More than 150,000 adults were randomly assigned to either have an annual chest X-ray for four years or not, and then they were followed for thirteen years to see how many were diagnosed with lung cancer and whether earlier diagnosis made a difference. What researchers found was that the rate of diagnosis of lung cancer was no different in the two groups and there was absolutely no difference in survival. Although chest X-rays don't expose you to very much radiation, why have any exposure if there is no benefit to your health? In addition, fifty-four people without lung cancer had complications, not from the X-ray, but from the biopsy that was done following an abnormal chest X-ray to see whether they did have cancer.

Another example is the routine urinalysis. This used to be part of the annual physical exam for everyone, beginning in childhood. One goal was to detect bacteria in the urine before it went on to infect the kidneys. While this has been shown to be beneficial in pregnant women, in other groups that is not the case. People who are routinely screened are more likely to end up on antibiotics for a prolonged period of time to kill the bacteria but no less likely to end up with a kidney infection. Why? It turns out that bacteria that are detected in asymptomatic nonpregnant people are not likely to cause a problem. In spite of this, some doctors still get the routine urinalysis.

My approach to testing is quite restrictive. I don't order laboratory tests unless they are part of a diagnostic work-up in someone who has symptoms or unless there is good evidence that routine testing in someone without symptoms has value. In children this means that I do screen for lead poisoning but I don't do a urinalysis. I have seen too often the consequences of unnecessary testing leading to more testing to figure out why the first test was wrong. That does the patient no good.

I do realize that in this regard, I am fighting a losing battle. A lot of people distrust doctors who are reluctant to order tests. Thankfully, an initiative led by the American Board of Internal Medicine Foundation, called Choosing Wisely, is under way to make it clear to doctors and patients which tests are being overused. They've been working with medical specialists to come up with a list of "Five Things Physicians and Patients Should Question" in their areas of expertise. On their lists: Annual EKGs for low-risk people; pap smears in women younger than twenty-one years; CT scans and MRIs in people who faint; and back X-rays in people with backaches.

While these efforts may not convince everyone that overtesting is a bad idea, at least it will let you know what the evidence (regardless of cost) says.

DR. B'S BOTTOM LINE:

It is natural for both doctors and their patients to want to "rule everything out" during a routine appointment. This is likely due to the natural motivation to want to catch any possible problem before it gets worse. And if the test finds nothing you get to breathe a sigh of relief. This, however, is neither a healthy nor an efficient practice. A doctor who overtests a patient is not doing that patient any favors—and he or she may even be exposing that patient to danger. Patients who demand tests from their doctors should realize that every test is a double-edged sword, and you could be in for much more cost and anguish than you bargained for.

64

IS THE INTERNET A GOOD PLACE TO GET MEDICAL INFORMATION?

When my friend and colleague *Good Morning America* anchor Robin Roberts was diagnosed with myelodysplastic syndrome (MDS) as a result of treatment she received years ago for breast cancer, I provided her with a lot of medical advice. One of the first things I said was "Don't Google it." MDS is a disorder of the bone marrow that can lead to leukemia. In fact, MDS used to be called pre-leukemia. However, it is mainly seen in people who are much older than Robin and not in nearly as good shape. I knew that even on reputable websites, the information she would see in terms of prognosis would be unnecessarily frightening and not relevant to her personally.

Her instinct to look online is the norm. The Internet is a potentially bottomless source of information on health. It is truly a game changer in terms of expanding your knowledge about your well-being. While medical personnel are still the first choice for most people with health concerns, according to data from the Pew Research Center's Internet & American Life Project, four out of five Americans who use the Internet have looked to it as a resource for health-related information. In many cases this is a good thing; searches on the Internet are already leading us to become more informed consumers of health care. However, like any powerful tool, the Internet can be dangerous if not used properly.

Here's when it's a good thing:

Research shows the Internet can empower you, which can enrich your relationship with your physician. Online sites can provide information about medical conditions and offer guidelines for treatment. That allows you to prepare questions for your appointments so you can have more in-depth conversations with your doctors. Knowing the facts in advance helps you to mentally process the alternatives for treatment before hearing them in the physician's office. This added time to think about options can allow you to become more involved in your own care plans and help you choose a treatment option that is best for you. It can also give you more confidence about your choices, knowing that you took ownership of your health care and were an active participant in it.

One of the best things about the Internet is the proliferation of online communities for people with various health conditions. This gives you—regardless of where you live, and how rare your medical condition—an opportunity to enter a "virtual" gathering place to gain information and support. Have a condition that has stigma attached? No problem. Online your identity can be secure. Want to know where new drug trials are taking place? Ask others with the same condition. I refer patients to online communities all the time.

Every week I host a Twitter chat called abcDrBchat, in which we have a conversation about one health topic. We've covered everything from cancer in young adults to finding treatments for rare diseases. During these exchanges disease experts, disease advocates, and patients share information and insights. We always include as one of the questions, "What are the best online sources for information and support?" In this way, people who are interested in learning more can go to sites that have been vetted. Online communities have become critical to the mental and physical health of people with chronic diseases.

Unfortunately, for all the good that the Internet provides in terms of access, there are also many pitfalls to be wary of. We all know by now that much of the medical information you read online is not vetted through the traditional editorial process for accuracy. It may be difficult for people without medical training to sort the wheat from the chaff when it comes to health information online without guidance. While the more search-savvy among us might see a big difference between a reputable site and one that is less than reliable, for all too many, these differences may not be as clear. Anyone with a computer can set up a website and post information. Having so much health content from uncredited and noncredentialed sources allows incomplete, misleading, and even totally incorrect information to be presented as fact. This is especially true when it comes to certain contentious topics in which myths and misconceptions endure despite scientific evidence to the contrary. Believing erroneous material might lead some people to distrust their doctor if the latter's advice is contrary to information recently gleaned.

In addition, the Internet is loaded with sites set up by unscrupulous people selling unproven and sometimes dangerous "cures" for untreatable diseases. These sites prey on the most vulnerable members of society. Unfortunately, it can be quite difficult to tell the difference between these websites and the legitimate ones.

DR. B'S BOTTOM LINE:

Overall, the Internet if used properly is a tremendous asset for promoting health. Nothing empowers patients more and gives them better control over their health decisions than knowledge. You just have to make sure you are getting credible information. Use what you learn online as a way of having a more informed dialogue with your doctor.

TIPS FOR FINDING CREDIBLE WEBSITES AND USING ONLINE INFORMATION

- Ask your doctor for recommendations. This is a great starting point and helps open a conversation.
- Begin with government websites. You know that these sites are unbiased and not linked to product sales. From there you can find other links to trusted nongovernmental sites. Some of my favorites are:
  - www.nih.gov: Info on any medical condition
  - www.cdc.gov: Info on all public health issues

- www.fda.gov: Info on drugs, medical products, food safety
- www.ahrq.gov: Info on what care you need.
- www.pubmed.gov: Search the published peer-reviewed literature.
- www.Healthfinder.gov: Online health encyclopedia with more than 1,600 topics.

- If you find a website that interests you, check it out at Health on the Net, www.HON.CH. It is an organization that accredits health websites based on certain ethical standards and helps you avoid scams.
- Use caution:
  - Never buy any medical product over the Internet without first talking to your doctor.
  - Never give personal medical information on the Internet.
  - Share the information you find with your doctor. It's a great way to know whether what you find applies to you.
- Consult these other helpful references for finding great health websites:
  - "Evaluating Online Sources of Health Information," National Cancer Institute, www.cancer.gov/cancertopics/cancerlibrary/health info online
  - "Trust It or Trash It?" www.trustortrash.org
  - Quackwatch, www.quackwatch.org.

65

ARE GENETIC TESTS EFFECTIVE?

Not long ago I did a story on a family that had spent nearly two hundred thousand dollars to sequence each family member's genome in its entirety. They were not your average family. The father worked for a company that does genomic sequencing and his daughter spent the summer working in a genetics lab. They viewed themselves as pioneers, peering into their own cells for clues to the diseases that might develop over the course of their lives. As I talked with them in their living room, the daughter combed through genetic sequences on her computer, trying to identify any genes that might be predictive of disease. Their goal: Early detection to improve prevention. They hoped their genomes would reveal the secrets of what lay ahead, so they could change their future.

Your genome is your complete genetic code. You inherit your DNA from your parents and your genes play a large role in your risk for developing many diseases. If you have the gene for Huntington's disease, you will develop the condition. End of story. For most diseases it isn't so simple. Whether you develop a disease will depend on your genetic predisposition and many environmental factors. The hope with genetic sequencing or genome mapping is that if you know what you are at greatest risk for, you can change your environment to reduce the chance that you will develop disease.

Through the family's analysis they discovered that both the father and daughter were at risk for blood clots forming, especially if they ate foods high in vitamin K. Based on these findings they decided to make some lifestyle changes. They stopped eating spinach, a vitamin K–rich food, and took special care when flying, a setting that raises your risk of developing blood clots. The daughter would opt to use a form of birth control other than the oral contraceptive pill since that can also raise the risk of blood clots. They viewed the genome mapping as a big success.

Entire genomic mapping is rarely done outside of research settings, due to the cost. But there are now direct-to-consumer genetic tests offered for as low as three hundred dollars. Think of them as "genomics lite." Although they are still in their infancy, many people find it hard to resist the lure of predicting their future risk of illness. But are these pricey tests worth it? Are the results a reliable predictor of what illnesses await?

In a word, no—or at least, not yet. Not only are these tests expensive, but they can be misleading and ultimately dangerous. Many consumers and even doctors don't have a complete understanding of the concept of risk that lies at the heart of these tests. Here is what I mean. For another story on ABC, I had my DNA analyzed by the Navigenics test kit. This kit is only available through doctor's offices and corporate wellness programs. The analysis gave me my risk as compared to the rest of the population for twenty-four different conditions. Results come in two colors, orange for those where your overall risk is greater than 25 percent *or* your risk is more than 20 percent above the average person for that condition, and gray, those conditions for which your risk is lower than that. Are you still with me? Here is what I found out: My risk of lupus, a severe autoimmune disorder, came up in orange. It was almost two and a half times the average risk. Sounds scary, right? Actually, even with that greater risk, the chance that over my lifetime I will *not* develop lupus is 99.93 percent. How can that be? Well, the chance that the average person will not develop lupus is 99.97 percent. So my risk of getting lupus is higher than most but clearly isn't something that I need to worry about. By the way, my producer had her blood tested, too. It said her risk of developing lupus was around 4 percent. Interesting, given that she already has lupus.

There were three other conditions—Crohn's disease, sarcoidosis, and multiple sclerosis—that all came up in orange. Again, for all these diseases my lifetime chance of *not* getting them was still around 99 percent or better. Without a good understanding of risk, I might have found the labels "above average risk" quite concerning.

Other results are disconcerting for different reasons. Based on my genetic markers, my lifetime risk of melanoma is only 2.3 percent, much lower than average. Now what do I do with this information? Do I stop using sunscreen and go back to using tanning oil like I did in high school?

Another big concern has to do with quality and reproducibility of the results. There is very little regulation of the direct-to-consumer genetic testing industry. In a scathing 2010 report by the U.S. Government Accountability Office, federal officials lambasted companies for providing misleading results, after officials reviewed the predictions from tests they had independently sent out. Investigators purchased ten test kits from four different companies. They then had five volunteers send two samples to each company. They found that the participants often received different risk information across the four companies. One individual was told he was at below-average, average, and above-average risk for high blood pressure and prostate cancer. None of the companies could provide complete risk information for an African-American participant, due to limited data in their systems, but none disclosed this before the kits were purchased.

So with all of these troubling issues in mind, is there a better way for individuals to get an accurate idea of their particular risk profiles while avoiding the potential pitfalls of these tests? It turns out there is—and not only has it has been available to us all along, but it's *free* and it is underutilized. It's knowing your family history.

When it comes to many conditions—particularly chronic conditions—the simple act of taking a family history trumps genetic testing for a number of reasons. Not the least of these is the fact that while a genetic test explores only the biological/hereditary basis for disease, family history can capture a much more holistic set of variables, including environment and behavioral norms. If there is a disease that runs in your family—your father had it, so did his father and mother, and his brother as well—you don't need an analysis of your genome to tell you that you had better pay attention to that one. If obesity runs in your family, who cares whether your genome says your risk is higher or lower than the general population's? Some combination of genetics and environment (how your family eats and exercises) is probably setting you up for weight gain.

I know what you may be thinking. What about the family I told you about earlier that found out that they were at increased risk for blood clots? Turns out that the father had two relatives who had problems with clots at a young age. A good family history would have easily picked that up and they then could have asked to be specifically tested for that clotting defect. Would have cost a lot less than two hundred grand.

I am not averse to genetic testing. There are circumstances where it can be very useful. Women who have a family history of early breast and ovarian cancer should speak to their doctors about whether getting tested for the BRCA genes makes sense. People with early onset of Alzheimer's disease in their families may want to get tested to see if they carry genes putting them at increased risk. Couples planning on having children can learn whether they are carriers for many devastating genetic diseases, such as Tay-Sachs. People going on certain medications can get testing to see how their bodies will metabolize them. The future of genomics to improve our ability to provide individualized advice and treatment is incredible, but at this time still limited.

DR. B'S BOTTOM LINE:

While certainly not as high-tech and sexy as genomic mapping, relying on the tried-and-true approach of family history is the best way to predict your future health risks. Your family history can help you and your doctor take precautions to keep you healthy. As genetic tests become more advanced and more specific in the years to come, it is entirely likely that they will play a larger part in the decisions we make regarding our health.

TELLING YOUR FAMILY HEALTH STORY

The surgeon general of the United States declared Thanksgiving to also be National Family History Day. What could be easier after a big turkey dinner than to pull out your family history form and get some information? The next time you have a family get-together, take a few minutes to talk about and to write down any health problems that seem to run in your family. Learning about your family's health history may help ensure a longer, healthier future together. It may even save your life.

Here are links to a few online tools to track your history:

- "Adult Family History Form" (American Medical Association), www.ama-assn.org/resources/doc/genetics/adult_history.pdf.
- "My Family Health Portrait: A Tool from the Surgeon General," www.familyhistory.hhs.gov/fhh-web/home.action.

66

DOES A PSA TEST ACCURATELY DETECT PROSTATE CANCER?

In 1980, my mother-in-law, Bert, went in for a breast biopsy. Luckily, the lump was benign. Before she had a chance to celebrate, the doctor called her with some bad news. The lab had found dispersed cancer cells in the surrounding area, which could eventually form a tumor. Bert, always cautious, opted for a radical mastectomy. There was no other option for her. She couldn't live with what she termed "a ticking time bomb." At the time, she didn't realize that cancer cells could live dormant in her body for her whole life. Years later, when she reflected back, she questioned her decision to have disfiguring surgery.

This debate of whether to "wait and see" still exists, especially with advancements in testing making it easier to locate cancer cells in the earliest stages. Nowhere is this more evident than with prostate screening. In recent years there have been few debates within the cancer community that have been as vigorous and contentious as cancer marker screening through blood tests. For men, the most contested test is for elevated levels of PSA, or prostate-specific antigen, in the blood. PSA is a specific type of protein that is made by the prostate, and unusually high levels of this substance in the blood have been seen with prostate cancer.

When PSA was initially developed as a test, its use was pretty specific. It was designed for use in men who had been treated for prostate cancer to see if their cancer was coming back. A rising PSA in a man who had undergone prostate surgery indicated that the treatment wasn't totally successful. In 1994, this test began to be used in otherwise healthy men to look for early signs of prostate cancer.

It is impossible to hear the word *cancer* without having a visceral reaction. It is a word that is often whispered rather than spoken loudly. The problem is that not all cancers are the same. There are cancers that kill quickly and cancers you can live with unknowingly without ever having any symptoms. Prostate cancer lies heavily in the latter category. We know this from autopsy studies of men who died from other causes. While it's rare to see it in men in their forties, it rises every decade after that. By the time a man hits his sixties the odds are you can find prostate cancer cells if you look hard enough.

A good cancer screening test should be able to detect cancer cells that are going to do harm, in a time frame that allows you to do something to prevent it. The problem is that PSA testing doesn't discriminate so well. It detects three kinds of prostate cancer. The first are cancers that may be growing so slowly that you will die with them, not from them. It also detects cancers that are so aggressive that even finding them early won't prevent illness. Lastly, it detects cancers that are going to do harm but through early detection can be totally treated. There is a big debate as to how many of the cancers that are detected through PSA testing fall into each of those three groups. But this much is clear: The benefit in terms of prolonging a man's life isn't very great.

Because of the inconclusive nature of PSA testing, the U.S. Preventive Services Task Force (USPSTF) published controversial recommendations calling for an end to routine PSA-based screening for prostate cancer. They found that the harm from detecting asymptomatic cancer outweighed the benefits. Here is why. The lifetime risk of getting prostate cancer is around 16 percent. The lifetime risk of dying of prostate cancer is around 3 percent. This means that most men who get prostate cancer don't die from it. The USPSTF looked at all the studies in which large numbers of men were randomly assigned to be screened or to get their usual care, to see what impact routine screening had on survival. Surprisingly, they didn't see much of an impact. At best, one prostate-cancer-related death was prevented for every one thousand men screened for ten years. Even worse, they saw no effect in terms of overall survival; these men were dying of something else. Overall, during the study period, death rates from any cause were no different in men who were screened for prostate cancer and those who weren't.

There's more to the story. If PSA-based screening were without harm, even the hint of a slight benefit might be worth talking about, but that is not the case. While the PSA test is a simple blood test, the next step for those with elevated values is a prostate biopsy. This carries risks for bleeding, infection, and urinary difficulties, in about one-third of men. If cancer is detected, since it can be difficult to determine how aggressive it is, more than 90 percent of men get treated with some combination of drug therapy, surgery, or radiation. These therapies have very high rates of side effects, principally sexual dysfunction and urinary incontinence.

Dr. Richard Albin, the scientist who discovered PSA, is in agreement with the USPSTF recommendation. In an opinion piece in the *New York Times* in 2010 he called the current use of PSA screening a "profit-driven public health disaster."

The American Cancer Society is equally skeptical that there is great benefit from PSA-based screening. However, given that there is no better test available, they recommend that an informed decision to screen should come out of a conversation between a man and his doctor about risks and benefits. This conversation should take place starting at age fifty for those at average risk and at forty-five for those at higher risk.

The American Urological Association, the group representing the doctors who treat prostate cancer, recommends that all men ages forty and above be offered PSA-based screening. They point to a decline in deaths from prostate cancer as proof that screening works. They find flaws in the clinical trials that show that screening large groups of men with PSA has no benefit.

It's clear the debate around PSA-based screening isn't over. The studies that have been done all have flaws that make firm conclusions hard to come by. However, my overall approach to testing, as I've mentioned throughout, is that we should never undertake a test unless there is very strong evidence that the benefits outweigh the harms. I have seen too many otherwise healthy people turned into patients after having tests they didn't need. You always hear about the patient who claims their life was saved because something was found incidentally on a routine blood test or X-ray. You don't hear as much about the patients whose lives were harmed in significant ways by having had unnecessary testing. We need to do a better job of sharing those stories too.

The USPSTF comes under fire whenever they recommend less testing, but it's important to have an unbiased group review evidence and make recommendations. They make it a point to not have anyone on the review who has a financial stake in the outcome.

DR. B'S BOTTOM LINE:

It is unfortunate, but the PSA test does not accurately distinguish between cancers that will kill you and those that are harmless. The decision to undergo any cancer screening test may seem deceptively simple—after all, who wouldn't want to get as much information as possible? But when it comes to PSA testing there is no one right decision. My advice: Get informed and have a conversation with your doctor about what you want to do, before your blood gets drawn.

67

SHOULD I GET DENTAL X-RAYS EVERY YEAR?

While I was employed at the CDC, like millions of Americans I had minimal dental insurance. The visit to the dentist—including cleaning, X-rays, and examination—would run me close to a couple of hundred dollars. I'd be lucky to get twenty bucks back from insurance. I learned firsthand that you pay closer attention to medical costs when the dollars come directly from your wallet. While my family continued to have our yearly dental checkups, when the question of X-rays came up, we'd always find a reason to push it off to the next year. It turns out we were inadvertently doing a good thing. While I had always believed that X-rays were a critical part of the annual dental exam, it turns out I was wrong.

With any medical test, the goal is to maximize the benefits and minimize the harms. The benefit from dental X-rays is the ability to detect dental disease that is not apparent to the naked eye at a time when an intervention can be made. The harm is exposure to ionizing radiation and the risk it poses over one's lifetime for developing cancer. Dentists tend to downplay these doses of radiation by comparing them to exposures from other factors in the environment, and, all told, radiation from dental X-rays is relatively low, especially compared to doses in decades past. But exposing ourselves and especially our children to *any* excess or unnecessary radiation should be a concern. The radiation from X-rays is cumulative, meaning that the damage to the genes from these and other sources of radiation can build up over time, slowly increasing the likelihood of alterations to our DNA that can lead to cancer.

So how do you protect yourself? Whenever a dentist wants to give you an X-ray, ask her or him if it is necessary or if there is another way to get the information. Perhaps you can you stretch out the interval between X-rays. I'm not alone in supporting this approach. It is actually what is suggested by the American Dental Association (ADA). They currently recommend X-rays every two to three years for healthy adults.

The ADA's long-standing position is that dentists should carefully examine the risk/benefit ratio and *only* order dental X-rays when they are needed for diagnosis and treatment, not on asymptomatic patients or automatically on a calendar basis. That's right, their own professional association recommends taking X-rays much less frequently than most dentists do.

Guidelines aside, technology has also evolved in such a way so that when you get an X-ray, you should be exposed to less radiation than in the past. One of these advancements has been the development of new faster E- and F-speed films, which require less radiation to give an accurate picture. But many dentists have been slow to upgrade to the faster speed film, with the slower D-speed film accounting for about 70 percent of the film used. Don't be afraid to ask your dentist which they use.

For those of you like me, with children in the orthodontic phase, take heed. Orthodontists are likely to recommend additional films as they monitor the progress of teeth shifting. Quite often, they will have even fancier scanning machines that emit even more radiation than conventional X-rays. Before agreeing to any films, take into consideration that your dentist might have recently taken some. If that is the case, get copies to share.

DR. B'S BOTTOM LINE:

Just as with any optional testing, before you automatically agree to X-rays, make sure that your dentist has explored all other options. Have them check when your last set was. If it's been less than two years, ask if it's really necessary. If your dentist does not adhere to the ADA guidelines, ask them to explain why. If their answer is not satisfactory, it may be time to find another dentist.

TIPS FROM THE FDA FOR REDUCING RADIATION EXPOSURE

- Ask your dentist how an X-ray will help. Is there some other way to get the same information?
- Don't refuse an X-ray. If your dentist feels it is important for the health of your teeth, don't say no. The risk from an individual X-ray is very small.
- Don't insist on an X-ray. If your dentist says you don't need one, don't demand one.
- Tell your dentist if you are pregnant. Best to avoid any X-rays until after you deliver.
- Ask if a protective shield can be used. You want to make sure the X-ray beam only goes where it is needed.
- Ask your dentist if he/she uses the faster (E- or F-speed) film for X-rays. This can provide high-quality images at lower radiation exposure.
- Know your X-ray history. Keep a record of your X-rays and take it with you if you go to a new dentist, orthodontist, or move. Why get a new X-ray if you just had one?

Source: Adapted from www.fda.gov/ForConsumers/ConsumerUpdates/ucm095505.htm.

68

ARE HOSPITALS MORE DANGEROUS IN JULY?

Watch the premiere episode of any TV drama set in a teaching hospital and you are likely to see one or two errors perpetrated by bright-eyed residents, physicians green to day-to-day hospital life. These eager newbies have yet to acquire the skills of their seasoned attendings, who rule the hospital with iron fists. By the end of the show, the resident physicians will have learned an important lesson in humility as their older and wiser colleagues rush in to save the patient, leaving the residents determined to improve and earn the respect of their colleagues.

I remember the first week of my pediatric residency. After four years of hitting the books and working on the wards under the direction of licensed doctors, I finally had "M.D." after my name and was going to start caring for patients on my own! My best friend from medical school, Mark, and I used to joke all the time that at some point someone was going to come up behind us, tap us on the shoulder, and call us out as the imposters we feared we were. "Excuse me, you are no doctor!" While that never happened, the early days of residency training are an incredibly stressful period in a young doctor's life. A time when you are trying to act like you really know what you are doing, when in reality, you don't even know how to log on to the computer.

While these are hard times for new doctors, what if *you* find yourself in the position of needing medical care in July, when fresh med school graduates transition from the classroom to the hospital? Should you delay elective surgery? Should you avoid teaching hospitals? It is a question that a number of studies have sought to answer, and while media coverage has focused on those studies that show an increased risk, the research appears to fall on both sides of the fence.

One of the best reviews of this question was published in 2011 in the *Annals of Internal Medicine*. The authors reviewed thirty-nine studies that looked into what has been called the "July Effect," the impact on patients' health of being in the hospital in July as compared to other times of the year. The studies came from several different countries, though most were from the United States. When looking at increased risk of death, half of the really good studies showed an increase and half did not. When it came to medical errors of various kinds, only five studies were felt to be of high quality and only one of these high-quality studies showed an increased rate of errors. Lastly, they looked at how efficiently the hospital worked: Things like length of stay, hospital charges, and how long operations took to complete. Here there were seven high-quality studies and again there was a split, with about half showing problems in July and half not.

Why are there so many conflicting studies? There are a number of reasons. This is a really hard thing to study. There is no uniform approach to patient care across all hospitals, so a study looking at one hospital really only tells you something about that hospital. In addition, the systems in place to capture medical errors are primitive and changing, so counting mistakes in many settings isn't very accurate. A recent report by the inspector general in the Department of Health and Human Services found that 86 percent of incidents involving harm to Medicare patients in hospitals went unreported. It is hard to measure small differences in how you are treated in the hospital in different months if most mistakes aren't even recorded.

However, I do have a personal take on this issue. Early in my career, I spent five years as the pediatric residency director at the University of California, San Diego. During those years when I was in charge of the trainees, the period that concerned me the most wasn't July; it was June. During July we watched the new interns and residents like hawks. They might have thought they were flying solo but they weren't. We put the best senior doctors on the wards and double- and triple-checked the orders that were being written. In June it was entirely different. Residents were seasoned, they knew what they were doing, and our focus was on the upcoming transition. In June, some residents got a bit sloppy. Those who were leaving for jobs had their minds elsewhere. The interns who were just finishing up their first grueling year of training were exhausted and looking forward to no longer being the low ones on the totem pole.

Clearly, though, the message that the public receives with regard to this "July Effect" skews in the more interesting of the two possible directions. A nonscientific review of the media coverage of this phenomenon using a Google search revealed that popular news sites and other media sources were far more likely to report that this effect exists than they were to acknowledge research to the contrary. It may be that reading about what will kill us is much more interesting than finding out what is not likely to! But whatever the reason, it is easy to see how this lack of balance may shape the perceptions of the public in general.

DR. B'S BOTTOM LINE:

The data are mixed, but if anything can be shown, it is that while the month might make a bit of difference, it is not the primary determinant of your chances of making it out of the hospital alive should you require hospital-based care. The important thing is that you get the care you need, whenever it is you may need it. Enter the hospital on your guard and follow my tips for hospital safety. This is a good idea no matter what month it is.

TOP TEN QUESTIONS TO ASK WHEN YOU ARE IN THE HOSPITAL

1. WHY IS THIS TEST BEING DONE?

Before having any test, understand its purpose and find out how the results will affect your care. Especially if it is an invasive procedure, ask if there are any risks from the test itself and if so, if there is another way to get the information needed.

2. WHAT ARE THE RESULTS OF MY TESTS?

If you had tests done, ask for the results and for someone to go over them with you so you understand them. Request a written copy of results to keep with your medical records.

3. HAVE YOU WASHED YOUR HANDS?

Before anyone touches you, ask, "Have you washed your hands?" It may be hard to do, but it could prevent a life-threatening infection.

4. WHO WILL BE TAKING CARE OF ME?

Your team can include the head doctor (also called an "attending"), fellows, residents, medical students, nurse practitioners, nurses, and nursing assistants. It can be very confusing. Ask for, or keep, a list of who is providing your care. Just like in baseball, it's hard to keep track without a program!

5. WHEN WILL MY TUBES BE REMOVED?

If you have any tubes coming into your body (IV, urinary catheter), ask when they can be taken out. This will reduce the chances that you will get an infection.

6. WHAT ARE THE MEDICATIONS I'M TAKING?

Ask for a list of all the medications that they are going to be giving you and have the nurse tell you what each is for. Pain medicines, sleeping pills, and stool softeners are often prescribed on an "as-needed" basis. You are in the driver's seat as to whether you want these. The fewer medicines you take, the fewer side effects you will experience.

7. WHO IS PERFORMING MY OPERATION?

Before having surgery, ask who will be doing it and exactly what will be done. You have the right to know whether your surgery will be performed by the head of your medical team or a resident. If you aren't comfortable with the answer, ask to speak to the head of the team.

8. ARE THERE ANY SUPPORT SERVICES FOR PATIENTS?

Many hospitals have integrative or complementary health departments that offer all kinds of programs, from bedside yoga to nutritional counseling. These can be a tremendous support to your emotional health.

9. COULD YOU EXPLAIN THAT AGAIN?

Some health care providers can forget that you may not have a medical degree! Medical terminology that seems obvious to someone working in a hospital is like a foreign language to most patients. Keep asking for things to be clarified if you don't understand exactly what they mean.

10. WHEN CAN I GO HOME?

While a hospital is a great place to be when you need to be there, getting out as soon as you can is also important. Fewer days in the hospital means less time for you to pick up something you didn't come in with.

CONCLUSION

Throughout this book I've been leaving you with my Bottom Line to help you safely navigate confusing medical decisions. I truly believe staying healthy is really pretty simple—not necessarily easy, but definitely not complicated.

I know it can be hard to get answers you can trust. Hopefully, if you follow my advice you will understand the principles of good health, from how good nutrition and staying physically and mentally active can set you on the path toward a longer life, to bigger concerns like how to find a doctor you can really talk with and what to do when illness strikes. They will, in turn, help you make better decisions about your well-being.

Throughout this book, my only goal has been to provide information that will empower you to improve your health. I also hope the advice I have provided helps you become a more educated consumer, especially when it comes to spending your money on products with claims that are too good to be true. Not only am I not trying to sell you anything, but much of the advice I'm giving you will save you money. There are a lot of things you invest in with the hopes of better health that simply don't deliver. Even though someone else is taking something, it doesn't mean it's right for you. When it comes to managing your care, don't be afraid to question why something you might not need is being prescribed or why a test is being recommended. Conversely, if you don't think you are getting adequate care, don't be afraid to stand up for yourself and have your physicians explain why they did not choose a particular treatment.

Remember, you can always find me on the air and online. If you've got something on your mind, I'm sure there are thousands of people with a similar question. I'll do my best to address it on one of our programs, on Facebook, or during one of my weekly Twitter chats. You'll find those by following me on Twitter at @DrRichardBesser or on Facebook at Dr. Richard Besser.

I leave you with my top ten Dr. B's Bottom Line list. These are the most important actions that you can do to stay healthy. Maintaining health is a lifelong commitment; it doesn't happen all at once. Pick one thing and make a small change toward a longer and healthier life. Then pick another and another. Before you know it you will be reaping the rewards. And that's the truth.

1. Eat a high-fiber, low-fat diet based primarily on plants.
   Remember, there are no bad foods, just those to eat in moderation.
2. Make exercise and movement a part of your life.
3. Don't smoke.
4. Know your family history.
5. Get vaccinated.
6. Find a doctor you can trust, while you are healthy.
7. Get a second opinion if you are sick.
8. Have friends and keep social.
9. Get enough sleep.
10. Own your health. It's your body and your life.
    Decide what is important to you.

ACKNOWLEDGMENTS

I have a newfound respect for real writers. My wife, Jeanne, is one. She has written five cookbooks and countless food columns for the *Atlanta Journal-Constitution*. Over twenty years I have watched as she has churned out prose that was engaging, informative, intelligent, and funny, all on a deadline. I wasn't sure how she did it with such ease, and after working on this book it is even more of a mystery to me.

My biggest thanks and total appreciation go to Jeanne. She and I worked on this book together. It really has been a full partnership in every sense of the word, in the same way that our marriage and our tennis game are. Many of our friends who are couples really don't enjoy playing tennis together; Jeanne and I do. I know that if a ball is hit over her head (she is five foot two) it is my responsibility to get it (I am six foot six). That's just the way it is. In writing this book together, I knew that she was the professional and I was the novice. Whenever I had a turn of phrase that was a bit awkward, it was her responsibility to fix it. I could not have asked for a better writing partner or partner in life.

Next my thanks go to our boys, Alex and Jack. I hope that the approach to health that we've laid out in this book is something that is now ingrained in them through how our family lives our lives. We really do walk the walk. Thanks for their questions over our dinner table and their patience and understanding when my work has caused me to miss more than a few meals, and tolerance when I use stories from our home to illustrate medical points on the air.

Thanks to my parents, Ruth and Bill Besser, for always believing in me and giving me the confidence to try new things (including Brussels sprouts and career changes). To my older brothers, Mitch and Andy, who each in his own way is trying to change lives. What wonderful role models. To my sister, Karen, the performer in the family, who died at far too young an age from a medical error. She would have gotten such a kick out of what I do for a living. There are so many things I wish I could have told her.

There are many people who inspired me to write this book and whom I want to thank. First and foremost are the viewers at ABC News who continually reach out to me with their health questions and continually hold me accountable for what I say. When I say something that isn't clear or that they don't agree with, they let me know it on our website, on my Facebook page, through Twitter, on voice mail, and even occasionally through the U.S. Postal Service. They make sure that I am truly communicating about health rather than speaking jargon. I wanted to see if through a book, clearly written, I could expand on some of the issues I cover on the air, providing a bit more background to explain the recommendations that I make.

Next are the people I work with who hail me in the hall or on the set; the people who stop me on the street or on the subway, looking for an honest ear to help them sort through a health problem. I hope that this book provides you with some of the answers you were looking for.

I want to thank all the medical residents who come to spend a month working in the medical unit of ABC News, bringing an interest in both journalism and medical communications. You give me the opportunity to keep abreast of the latest findings in medicine, you help ensure that our stories are based on the best available science, and you provide me with the chance to continue my love of teaching health, prevention, epidemiology, and communication. Your questions and work make my reporting so much better.

This book never would have been completed nor been as well informed without the terrific research assistance from Dan Childs, head of the ABC News medical unit, and Peg Rosen, a wonderful medical writer in Montclair, New Jersey. Dan has taught me so much about what an audience is looking for in medical coverage.

Three years ago I was working at the CDC when I got an email out of the blue from Amy Entelis, then head of talent at ABC News. She liked the way I was handling press conferences during the H1N1 pandemic and wanted to know if I had ever thought about being an on-air medical correspondent. She helped to broaden my concept of what it means to practice public health. A big thanks to Amy and to David Westin, who was president of ABC News at the time, for taking a chance on a true novice and letting me try to practice public health in front of a camera.

Thanks so much to Ben Sherwood, president of ABC News, and all the leadership there for continuing to support me on the air and especially to Ben for encouraging me to expand my reach and build my audience. To Eric Avram, who runs all of the units at ABC News and is the best boss anyone could ever hope for, thanks for supporting my growth on television and for helping me deal with the occasional culture shock.

I'd like to express my enormous gratitude to Diane Sawyer, who more than anyone has taught me how to communicate through the camera, how to try to convey the same feeling to millions of viewers that I do when I am sitting and talking one-on-one with a patient. Watching her make that connection every night is a privilege.

Big thanks to the following:

To Robin Roberts, who shows me every day the meaning of courage and the importance of sharing a bit of your heart with the audience, that it's okay to let them in. To George Stephanopoulos, for letting me see that you can be smart and still get silly every once in a while. What a pleasure it is to talk to you both about health on *GMA*.

To the other anchors at ABC News whom I get to sit and talk health with: David Muir, Dan Harris, Bianna Golodryga, Josh Elliott, and Lara Spencer.

To the producers who have been teaching me about the craft of making television, thanks so much for your patience and care: Ann Reynolds, Gitika Ahuja, Lana Zak, Cathy Becker, Tom Johnson, Susan Schwartz, Alice Maggin, and Diane Mendez.

To Roger Sergel, who ran the medical unit with such professionalism for so many years and taught me so much about medical journalism.

To the executive producers who every day see the importance of providing intelligent health information to our viewers: Tom Cibrowski, Chris Vlasto, Michael Corn, Jeanmarie Condon, and James Goldston.

To Kris Sebastian and Mimi Gurbst, who welcomed me with open arms when I first came to ABC News and helped me understand how a television news division operates. Your friendship made the transition possible.

To Mollie Riegger, the best assistant anyone could hope for, who does such a terrific job keeping me organized and being my sounding board.

To Teri Whitcraft, who led the charge on our global health initiative, Be the Change: Save a Life, and kept me invigorated and focused when my instinct was to lose hope.

To Patrick Alemi, who does my hair and challenges my politics.

To my alphabet soup full of friends and colleagues at the CDC, NIH, FDA, USDA, EPA, and the AHRQ, who work every day to protect the health of Americans and people around the globe. What a selfless group of public servants.

To Matt Inman, my editor at Hyperion, for his keen eye and his guidance on how to explain things without the medical jargon that is my fallback. He has made this book so much better through his careful editing.

To Bob Barnett for his friendship and guidance. Without Bob, I would have been totally lost entering the media world.

Lastly, to my friends Mark Schechter and Phil Navin for their nightly reviews of my reporting (and wardrobe) on *Good Morning America* and *World News*.

NOTES

Chapter 1: Drop That French Fry and No One Gets Hurt: Your Questions on Diets, Nutrition, and Food Safety

1. Are Diets the Best Way to Lose Weight?
- Michael Pollan, "Unhappy Meals," *New York Times Magazine*, January 28, 2007, accessed November 4, 2012, www.nytimes.com/2007/01/28/magazine/28nutritionism.t.html.
- "Adult Obesity Facts," Centers for Disease Control and Prevention, last modified August 13, 2012, accessed September 10, 2012, www.cdc.gov/obesity/data/adult.html.
- "Childhood Obesity Facts," Centers for Disease Control and Prevention, last modified June 7, 2012, accessed September 10, 2012, www.cdc.gov/healthyyouth/obesity/facts.htm.
- "Celebrity Diets Debunked," *Good Morning America*, ABC News, February 12, 2011, abcnews.go.com/GMA/video/celebrity-diets-debunked-12900796.

2. Will Eating Six Small Meals a Day Instead of Three Big Ones Help Me Lose Weight?
- Sylvia M. O. Titan et al., "Frequency of Eating and Concentrations of Serum Cholesterol in the Norfolk Population of the European Prospective Investigation into Cancer (EPIC-Norfolk): Cross Sectional Study," *British Medical Journal* 323 (December 1, 2001): 1286–88.
- Jameason D. Cameron, Marie-Josée Cyra, and Éric Doucet, "Increased Meal Frequency Does Not Promote Greater Weight Loss in Subjects Who Were Prescribed an 8-Week Equi-Energetic Energy-Restricted Diet," *British Journal of Nutrition* 103 (April 2010):1098–1101.
- Cara B. Ebbeling et al., "Effects of Dietary Composition on Energy Expenditure During Weight-Loss Maintenance," *Journal of the American Medical Association* 307 (June 27, 2012): 2627–34.

3. Are Juice Fasts Good for Me?
- "Staying Away from Fad Diets," It's About Eating Right, Academy of Nutrition and Dietetics, accessed September 10, 2012, www.eatright.org/public/content.aspx?id=6851#.UD6MDmjhd1Y.

4. Can Eating Too Much Sugar Cause Diabetes?

- Press Release, "Number of Americans with Diabetes Rises to Nearly 26 Million," Centers for Disease Control and Prevention, January 26, 2011, www.cdc.gov/media/releases/2011/p0126_diabetes.html.
- Press Release, "Number of Americans with Diabetes Projected to Double or Triple by 2050," Centers for Disease Control and Prevention, October 22, 2010, www.cdc.gov/media/pressrel/2010/r101022.html.
- "Diabetes Statistics," American Diabetes Association, data from the 2011 National Diabetes Fact Sheet (released January 26, 2011), accessed September 10, 2012, www.diabetes.org/diabetes-basics/diabetes-statistics.
- "Diabetes Myths," American Diabetes Association, accessed September 10, 2012, www.diabetes.org/diabetes-basics/diabetes-myths.
- "Type 1 Diabetes," *A.D.A.M. Encyclopedia,* PubMed Health, review date June 28, 2011, accessed September 10, 2012, www.ncbi.nlm.nih.gov/pubmedhealth/PMH0001350.
- "Type 2 Diabetes," *A.D.A.M. Encyclopedia,* PubMed Health, review date June 28, 2011, accessed September 10, 2012, www.ncbi.nlm.nih.gov/pubmedhealth/PMH0001356.
- "What Is Diabetes?," Diabetes Research Wellness Foundation, accessed September 10, 2012, www.diabeteswellness.net/Portals/0/files/DRWFUSdiabetes.pdf.
- "National Diabetes Statistics, 2011," National Diabetes Information Clearinghouse, last modified December 6, 2011, accessed June 2, 2012, www.diabetes.niddk.nih.gov/dm/pubs/statistics/index.aspx.

5. Should I Drink Eight Glasses of Water a Day?

- Institute of Medicine. Panel on Dietary Reference Intakes for Electrolytes and Water, *Dietary Reference Intakes: Water, Potassium, Sodium, Chloride, and Sulfate* (Washington, DC: National Academies Press, 2005), www.iom.edu/Reports/2004/Dietary-Reference-Intakes-Water-Potassium-Sodium-Chloride-and-Sulfate.aspx.
- Michelle P. B. Guppy, Sharon M. Mickan, and Chris B. Del Mar, " 'Drink Plenty of Fluids': A Systematic Review of Evidence for This Recommendation in Acute Respiratory Infections," *British Medical Journal* 328 (February 26, 2004): 499–500.

6. Will Skipping Breakfast Help Me Lose Weight?

- "Build a Healthy Meal: 10 Tips for Healthy Meals," U.S. Department of Agriculture Center for Nutrition Policy and Promotion, DG TipSheet No. 7, June 2011, accessed September 10, 2011, www.choosemyplate.gov/food-groups/downloads/TenTips/DGTipsheet7BuildAHealthyMeal.pdf.
- "Putting the Fast in Breakfast—3 Quick and Easy Solutions," International Food Information Council Foundation, created January 2009, accessed September 10, 2012, www.foodinsight.org/LinkClick.aspx?fileticket=HvIhQAA0%2f0k%3d&tabid=1348.

7. Is Bottled Water Better than Tap?

- "Where You Live: Your Drinking Water Quality Reports Online," Consumer Confidence Reports, U.S. Environmental Protection Agency, last modified September 10, 2012, accessed September 10, 2012, water.epa.gov/lawsregs/rulesregs/sdwa/ccr/index.cfm.
- "2008 Water Fluoridation Statistics," Community Water Fluoridation, Centers for Disease

Control and Prevention, last modified October 22, 2010, accessed September 10, 2012, www
.cdc.gov/fluoridation/statistics/2008stats.htm.

- Nneka Leiba, Sean Gray, and Jane Houlihan, "2011 Bottled Water Scorecard," Environmental Working Group 2011, static.ewg.org/reports/2010/bottledwater2010/pdf/2011-bottled
water-scorecard-report.pdf.
- U.S. Government Accountability Office, "FDA Safety and Consumer Protections Are Often
Less Stringent than Comparable EPA Protections for Tap Water," 2009, accessed September
12, 2012, www.gao.gov/products/GAO-09-610.
- John G. Rodwan Jr., "Bottled Water 2011: The Recovery Continues," *Bottled Water Reporter*
52 (April/May 2012): 12–14, www.nxtbook.com/ygsreprints/IBWA/g25762_ibwa_bwr
_aprmay2012/#/16.
- U.S. Government Accountability Office, "Safe Drinking Water Act: Improvements in
Implementation are Needed to Better Assure the Public of Safe Drinking Water," Testimony
Before the Committee on Environment and Public Works, U.S. Senate, Statement of David
C. Trimble, Director, Natural Resources and Environment, 2011, accessed September 12,
2012, www.gao.gov/assets/130/126572.pdf.
- U.S. Government Accountability Office, "Drinking Water: Unreliable State Data Limit
EPA's Ability to Target Enforcement Priorities and Communicate Water Systems' Perfor-
mance," 2011, accessed September 12, 2012, www.gao.gov/assets/320/319780.pdf.
- Environmental Protection Agency, "Water Health Series: Filtration Facts," September 2005,
www.epa.gov/ogwdw/faq/pdfs/fs_healthseries_filtration.pdf.

8. Does Eating Eggs Give Me High Cholesterol?

- U.S. Department of Agriculture and U.S. Department of Health and Human Services,
Dietary Guidelines for Americans, 2010, 7th ed. (Washington, DC: U.S. Government Printing
Office, 2010), www.health.gov/dietaryguidelines/dga2010/dietaryguidelines2010.pdf.

9. Do I Need to Wash Prewashed Lettuce Mixes?

- "How Clean Is Bagged Salad?," ConsumerReports.org, last modified March 2010, accessed
September 12, 2012, www.consumerreports.org/cro/2012/05/how-clean-is-bagged-salad
/index.htm.
- "Raw Produce: Selecting and Serving It Safely," Food Facts from the U.S. Food and Drug
Administration, last modified April 5, 2012, accessed September 12, 2012, www.fda.gov/Food
/ResourcesForYou/Consumers/ucm114299.
- "Food Safety Practices," California Leafy Green Products Handler Marketing Agreement,
accessed September 12, 2012, www.caleafygreens.ca.gov/food-safety-practices.

10. Should I Rinse Chicken Before Cooking It?

- "Questions and Answers about Foodborne Illness (sometimes called 'Food Poisoning')),"
Centers for Disease Control and Prevention, last modified April 18, 2012, accessed September
12, 2012, www.cdc.gov/foodsafety/facts.html.
- "Foodborne Illness and Disease: Salmonella Questions and Answers," U.S. Department of
Agriculture, Food Safety and Inspection Service, last modified May 25, 2011, accessed
September 12, 2012, www.fsis.usda.gov/Factsheets/Salmonella_Questions_&_Answers/index
.asp.

Chapter 2: On Your Mark, Get Set, Move! Your Questions on Exercise, Fitness, and Sports Performance

15. Can I Be Fat and Fit?

- "Adult Obesity Facts," Centers for Disease Control and Prevention, last modified August 13, 2012, accessed September 10, 2012, www.cdc.gov/obesity/data/adult.html.
- "About BMI for Adults," Centers for Disease Control and Prevention, last modified September 13, 2011, accessed September 13, 2012, www.cdc.gov/healthyweight/assessing/bmi /adult_bmi/index.html.
- "Adult BMI Calculator: English," Centers for Disease Control and Prevention, last modified May 4, 2011, accessed September 10, 2012, www.cdc.gov/healthyweight/assessing/bmi/adult _bmi/english_bmi_calculator/bmi_calculator.html.

16. Should I Push Myself When Exercising—No Pain, No Gain?

- "Measuring Physical Activity Intensity," Centers for Disease Control and Prevention, last modified December 1, 2011, accessed September 13, 2012, www.cdc.gov/physicalactivity /everyone/measuring/index.html.
- "How Much Physical Activity Do You Need?" Centers for Disease Control and Prevention, last modified March 30, 2011, accessed September 13, 2012, www.cdc.gov/physicalactivity /everyone/guidelines/index.html.

17. If I'm Exercising, Should I Drink Sports Drinks?

- "Sports Drink Sales Get into Shape," *Beverage Industry* (online), July 12, 2011, accessed September 13, 2012, www.bevindustry.com/articles/84828-sports-drink-sales-get-into-shape.
- "Position Statement and Recommendations for Hydration to Minimize the Risk for Dehydration and Heat Illness," National Federation of State High School Associations (NFHS) Sports Medicine Advisory Committee (SMAC), revised and approved April 2008, accessed September 13, 2012, www.schsl.org/2010/Heat1.pdf.
- "How Sweet Is It? Calories and Teaspoons of Sugar in 12 Ounces of Each Beverage," Nutrition Source, Harvard School of Public Health 2009, accessed September 13, 2012, www .hsph.harvard.edu/nutritionsource/files/how-sweet-is-it-color.pdf.
- American Academy of Pediatrics, Committee on Nutrition and the Council on Sports Medicine and Fitness, "Sports Drinks and Energy Drinks for Children and Adolescents: Are They Appropriate?," *Pediatrics* 127 (June 1, 2011):1182–89.

18. Do I Need Thirty Minutes of Exercise a Day to Stay Healthy?

- Chi Pang Wen et al., "Minimum Amount of Physical Activity for Reduced Mortality and Extended Life Expectancy: A Prospective Cohort Study," *Lancet* 378 (October 1, 2011): 1244–53.
- "State Indicator Report on Physical Activity, 2010, National Action Guide," Centers for Disease Control and Prevention, accessed September 13, 2012, www.cdc.gov/physicalactivity /downloads/PA_State_Indicator_Report_2010_Action_Guide.pdf.

19. To Lose Weight, Is Exercise More Important than Diet?

- "Active at Any Size," National Institutes of Health, Weight-Control Information Network, NIH Publication No. 10-4352, last modified February 2010, accessed September 13, 2012, win.niddk.nih.gov/publications/active.htm#active.
- "Physical Activity for a Healthy Weight," Centers for Disease Control and Prevention, last modified September 13, 2011, accessed September 13, 2012.

20. Is Morning the Best Time to Exercise?

- Elizabeth Mendes, "Americans Get Back to Exercising in 2010," Gallup Wellbeing, May 27, 2010, accessed September 13, 2012, www.gallup.com/poll/137612/americans-back-exercising -often-2010.aspx.

21. Should I Stretch Before Exercising?

- Daniel Pereles, Alan Roth, and Darby J. S. Thompson, "A Large, Randomized, Prospective Study of the Impact of a Pre-Run Stretch on the Risk of Injury in Teenage and Older Runners," USA Track and Field Association, August 20, 2010, accessed September 13, 2012, www.usatf.org/stretchStudy/StretchStudyReport.pdf.

22. Will Wearing Ion or Magnetic Jewelry Improve My Sports Performance?

- "Product Info," Ionic Touch Negative Ion Bands, accessed October 4, 2012, ionictouch.com /product-info.htm.
- "Ion Bracelets and Ion Necklaces," Ki Flow, accessed October 4, 2012, kiflow.com.
- Press release, "Appeals Court Affirms Ruling in FTC's Favor in Q-Ray Bracelet Case," Federal Trade Commission, last modified June 24, 2011, accessed October 4, 2012, ftc.gov /opa/2008/01/qray.shtm.
- "Magnetic Therapy," American Cancer Society, last modified November 1, 2008, accessed October 4, 2012, www.cancer.org/Treatment/TreatmentsandSideEffects/Complementaryand AlternativeMedicine/ManualHealingandPhysicalTouch/magnetic-therapy.
- "Get the Facts: Magnets for Pain," National Center for Complementary and Alternative Medicine, last modified February 2012, accessed October 4, 2012, nccam.nih.gov/health /magnet/magnetsforpain.htm.

Chapter 3:   Oh Doctor, One More Thing! Your Questions When I'm Walking Out the Door

23. Will Counting Sheep Help Cure My Insomnia?

- Press release, "Longer Work Days Leave Americans Nodding Off on the Job," National Sleep Foundation, March 3, 2008, accessed October 4, 2012, www.sleepfoundation.org/article /press-release/longer-work-days-leave-americans-nodding-the-job.
- National Institutes of Health, "National Institutes of Health Sleep Disorders Research Plan," November 2011, NIH Publication No. 11-7820, www.nhlbi.nih.gov/health/prof/sleep /201101011NationalSleepDisordersResearchPlanDHHSPublication11-7820.pdf.

- Allison Harvey and Suzanna Payne, "The Management of Unwanted Pre-Sleep Thoughts in Insomnia: Distraction with Imagery Versus General Distraction," *Behaviour Research and Therapy* 40 (March 2002): 267–77.
- Julia Nelson and Allison Harvey, "Pre-Sleep Imagery Under the Microscope: A Comparison of Patients with Insomnia and Good Sleepers," *Behaviour Research and Therapy* 41 (March 2003): 273–84.
- Julia Nelson and Allison Harvey, "An Exploration of Pre-Sleep Cognitive Activity in Insomnia: Imagery and Verbal Thought," *British Journal of Clinical Psychology* 42 (September 2003): 271–88.
- "Healthy Sleep Tips," National Sleep Foundation, accessed October 4, 2012, www.sleep foundation.org/article/sleep-topics/healthy-sleep-tips.

24. Can I Make Up for Lack of Sleep During the Week by Sleeping Late on Weekends?

- "Healthy Sleep Tips," National Sleep Foundation, accessed October 4, 2012, www.sleep foundation.org/article/sleep-topics/healthy-sleep-tips.
- Gregory Belenky et al., "Patterns of Performance Degradation and Restoration During Sleep Restriction and Subsequent Recovery: A Sleep Dose-Response Study," *Journal of Sleep Research* 12 (March 2003): 1–12.
- "Sleep and Sleep Disorders: Fact Sheets," Centers for Disease Control and Prevention, last modified March 1, 2012, accessed October 4, 2012.www.cdc.gov/sleep/publications/factsheets .htm.
- "Healthy People 2020: Sleep Health," U.S. Department of Health and Human Services, last modified September 6, 2012, accessed October 4, 2012. www.healthypeople.gov/2020/ topicsobjectives2020/overview.aspx?topicId=38.
- Institute of Medicine, Committee on Sleep Medicine and Research, Board on Health Sciences Policy, *Sleep Disorders and Sleep Deprivation: An Unmet Public Health Problem* (Washington, DC: National Academics Press, 2006), www.iom.edu/~/media/Files/Report %20Files/2006/Sleep-Disorders-and-Sleep-Deprivation-An-Unmet-Public-Health-Problem /Sleepforweb.ashx.

25. Is Owning a Pet Good for My Health?

- "Be a Responsible Dog Owner," American Kennel Club, accessed October 4, 2012, www.akc .org/public_education/responsible_dog_owner.cfm.
- Harold Herzog, "The Impact of Pets on Human Health and Psychological Well-Being: Fact, Fiction, or Hypothesis?," *Current Directions in Psychological Science* 20 (August 2011): 236–39.
- "Home and Recreation Safety: Dog Bite Fact Sheet," Centers for Disease Control and Prevention, last modified April 1, 2008, accessed October 4, 2012, www.cdc.gov/Homeand RecreationalSafety/Dog-Bites/dogbite-factsheet.html.
- "Diseases from Dogs," Centers for Disease Control and Prevention, last modified February 8, 2011, accessed October 4, 2012, www.cdc.gov/healthypets/animals/dogs.htm.
- "Diseases from Cats," Centers for Disease Control and Prevention, last modified July 28, 2010, accessed October 4, 2012, www.cdc.gov/healthypets/animals/cats.htm.

- NIH News in Health, "Can Pets Help Keep You Healthy?," National Institutes of Health, February 2009, accessed October 4, 2012, newsinhealth.nih.gov/2009/February/feature1.htm.

26. Will Eating Dinner Together Make My Family Healthier?

- "The Importance of Family Dinners VI," National Center on Addiction and Substance Abuse at Columbia University, September 2010, www.casacolumbia.org/upload/2010/20100922familydinners6.pdf.

27. Will Doing Puzzles Prevent Alzheimer's Disease?

- "About Alzheimer's: Definition of Alzheimer's," Alzheimer's Foundation of America, accessed October 4, 2012, www.alzfdn.org/AboutAlzheimers/definition.html.
- "2012 Alzheimer's Disease Facts and Figures," Alzheimer's Association, March 2012, accessed October 4, 2012, www.alz.org/documents_custom/2012_facts_figures_fact_sheet.pdf.
- Martha Daviglus et al., "National Institutes of Health State-of-the-Science Conference Statement: Preventing Alzheimer's Disease and Cognitive Decline," *NIH Consensus State-of-the-Science Statements* 27 (April 26–28, 2010): 1–30, consensus.nih.gov/2010/docs/alz/ALZ_Final_Statement.pdf.

28. Will Condoms Prevent Me from Getting Sexually Transmitted Diseases?

- "Condom Fact Sheet in Brief," Centers for Disease Control and Prevention, last modified April 11, 2011, accessed November 3, 2012, www.cdc.gov/condomeffectiveness/docs/Condom_fact_Sheet_in_Brief.pdf.
- *Condoms and Sexually Transmitted Diseases,* brochure, U.S. Food and Drug Administration, last modified July 22, 2010, accessed November 3, 2012, www.fda.gov/ForConsumers/byAudience/ForPatientAdvocates/HIVandAIDSActivities/ucm126372.htm.
- "STD Trends in the United States: 2010 National Data for Gonorrhea, Chlamydia, and Syphilis," Centers for Disease Control and Prevention, last modified November 17, 2011, accessed November 8, 2012, www.cdc.gov/std/stats10/trends.htm.
- "HIV/AIDS Among Persons Aged 50 and Older," Centers for Disease Control and Prevention, last modified February 28, 2008, accessed November 8, 2012, www.cdc.gov/hiv/topics/over50/resources/factsheets/over50.htm.
- "Sexually Transmitted Diseases—Interactive Data 1996–2009," Centers for Disease Control and Prevention, accessed November 8, 2012, wonder.cdc.gov/std-std-race-age.html.

29. Can Using an iPod Damage My Hearing?

- "How Loud Is Too Loud? How Long Is Too Long?," National Institutes of Health, October 2009, NIH Publication No. 09-6433, accessed November 3, 2009, www.noisyplanet.nidcd.nih.gov/info/Pages/howloud.aspx.
- "Noise-Induced Hearing Loss," National Institutes of Health, NIH Publication No. 97-4233, last modified October 2008, accessed November 3, 2012, www.nidcd.nih.gov/health/hearing/pages/noise.aspx.

30. Will Using a Higher-Number Sunscreen Keep Me from Burning?

- "Skin Cancer Prevention and Early Detection," American Cancer Society, last modified September 20, 2012, accessed November 3, 2012, www.cancer.org/acs/groups/cid/documents /webcontent/003184-pdf.pdf.
- "UVA Radiation—A Danger Outdoors and Indoors," Skin Cancer Foundation, 2012, accessed November 4, 2012, www.skincancer.org/prevention/uva-and-uvb/uva-radiation-a -danger-outdoors-and-indoors.
- "Sunscreens," American Academy of Dermatology, 2012, accessed November 4, 2012, www .aad.org/media-resources/stats-and-facts/prevention-and-care/sunscreens.
- "FDA Sheds Light on Sunscreens," U.S. Food and Drug Administration, last modified May 17, 2012, accessed November 4, 2012, www.fda.gov/forconsumers/consumerupdates /ucm258416.htm.
- "What You Need to Know About Melanoma and Other Skin Cancers," National Cancer Institute, NIH Publication No. 10-7625, posted January 11, 2011, accessed November 4, 2012, www.cancer.gov/cancertopics/wyntk/skin.

32. Is Religion Good for My Health?

- Douglas Martin, "Lester Breslow, Who Linked Healthy Habits and Long Life, Dies at 97," *New York Times,* www.nytimes.com/2012/04/15/health/lester-breslow-who-tied-good-habits -to-longevity-dies-at-97.html
- James E. Enstrom and Lester Breslow, "Lifestyle and Reduced Mortality Among Active California Mormons, 1980–2004," *Preventive Medicine* 46 (February 2008): 133–36, psychology .ucdavis.edu/Labs/PWT/Image/emmons/file/16_Sheldon_Chapter-16-1%5B1%5D.pdf.

33. Is Antibacterial Soap Better than Plain Soap?

- Sally F. Bloomfield et al., "The Effectiveness of Hand Hygiene Procedures in Reducing the Risks of Infections in Home and Community Settings," *American Journal of Infection Control* 35, Supplement (December 2007): S27–S64.
- Allison E. Aiello, Elaine L. Larson, and Stuart B. Levy, "Consumer Antibacterial Soaps: Effective or Just Risky?," *Clinical Infectious Diseases* 45, Supplement 2 (2007): S137–S147.
- *An Ounce of Prevention Keeps the Germs Away: Seven Keys to a Safe Healthier Home,* brochure, Centers for Disease Control and Prevention, last modified April 24, 2008, accessed November 4, 2012, www.cdc.gov/ounceofprevention/docs/oop_brochure_eng.pdf.
- Stephen P. Luby et al., "Effect of Intensive Hand Washing Promotion on Childhood Diarrhea in High Risk Communities in Pakistan: A Randomized Controlled Trial," *Journal of the American Medical Association* 291 (June 4, 2004): 2547–54.

34. How Do I Protect Myself from Germs?

- "Study Reveals Kitchen Is Germiest Place in the Home," NSF International, 2004, accessed November 4, 2012, www.nsf.org/consumer/newsroom/fact_top10_germiest_places.asp.
- *An Ounce of Prevention Keeps the Germs Away: Seven Keys to a Safer Healthier Home,* brochure Centers for Disease Control and Prevention, last modified April 24, 2008, accessed November 4, 2012, www.cdc.gov/ounceofprevention/docs/oop_brochure_eng.pdf.

35. Is a Drink or Two a Day Good for Me?

- "Alcoholic Beverages and Cardiovascular Disease," American Heart Association, last
  modified March 31, 2011, accessed November 4, 2012, www.heart.org/HEARTORG
  /GettingHealthy/NutritionCenter/Alcoholic-Beverages-and-Cardiovascular-Disease_UCM
  _305864_Article.jsp.
- "Alcohol Use and Health," Centers for Disease Control and Prevention, last modified October
  1, 2012, accessed November 4, 2012, www.cdc.gov/alcohol/fact-sheets/alcohol-use.htm/.

36. Do Adults Need Shots?

- "Recommended Immunization Schedules for Persons Aged 0 through 18 Years, United
  States, 2012," Centers for Disease Control and Prevention, accessed November 4, 2012, www
  .cdc.gov/vaccines/schedules/downloads/child/0-18yrs-11x17-fold-pr.pdf.
- "Adolescent and Adult Vaccine Quiz: What Vaccines Do You Need?," Centers for Disease
  Control and Prevention, last modified May 31, 2012, accessed November 4, 2012, www2a.cdc
  .gov/nip/adultImmSched.

Chapter 4: Medicine Cabinet: Friend or Foe? Your Questions on Vitamins, Supplements, and Medications

37. Should I Take a Daily Multivitamin?

- U.S. Preventive Services Task Force, "Routine Vitamin Supplementation to Prevent Cancer
  and Cardiovascular Disease: Recommendations and Rationale," June 2003, Agency for
  Healthcare Research and Quality, www.uspreventiveservicestaskforce.org/3rduspstf/vitamins
  /vitaminsrr.htm.
- "Dietary Supplement Fact Sheet: Multivitamin/Mineral Supplements," Office of Dietary
  Supplements, National Institutes of Health, last reviewed January 12, 2012, accessed
  November 8, 2012, ods.od.nih.gov/factsheets/MVMS-HealthProfessional.
- National Institutes of Health State-of-the-Science Panel, National Institutes of Health State-of-
  the-Science Conference Statement, "Multivitamin/Mineral Supplements and Chronic Disease
  Prevention," *American Journal of Clinical Nutrition* 85, supplement (January 2007): 257S–264S.
- Jaime Gahche et al., "Dietary Supplement Use Among U.S. Adults Has Increased Since
  NHANES III (1988–1994)," NCHS Data Brief, no. 61, National Center for Health Statistics,
  2011, www.cdc.gov/nchs/data/databriefs/db61.htm.

38. Will Taking Vitamin C Prevent Me from Getting a Cold?

- Harri Hemilä, Elizabeth Chalker, and Bob Douglas, "Vitamin C for Preventing and
  Treating the Common Cold," *Cochrane Database of Systematic Reviews,* 2007, Issue 3, Art.
  No. CD000980.

39. Should I Take a Daily Aspirin to Prevent a Heart Attack, Stroke, or Cancer?

- Catherine Dube et al., U.S. Preventive Services Task Force, "The Use of Aspirin for Primary
  Prevention of Colorectal Cancer: A Systematic Review Prepared for the U.S. Preventive
  Services Task Force," *Annals of Internal Medicine* 146 (March 6, 2007): 365–75.

- Rosie O'Donnell, "My Heart Attack," blog entry, rosie.com, August 20, 2012, accessed November 9, 2012, rosie.com/my-heart-attack/.
- U.S. Preventive Services Task Force, "Aspirin for the Prevention of Cardiovascular Disease: Recommendation Statement," AHRQ Publication No. 09-05129-EF-2, March 2009, www.uspreventiveservicestaskforce.org/uspstf09/aspirincvd/aspcvdrs.htm.
- "Aspirin and Heart Disease," American Heart Association, last modified March 30, 2012, accessed July 24, 2012, www.heart.org/HEARTORG/Conditions/HeartAttack/Prevention TreatmentofHeartAttack/Aspirin-and-Heart-Disease_UCM_321714_Article.jsp.
- "Recommendations of Aspirin for Prevention of Cardiovascular Disease," Centers for Disease Control and Prevention, last modified September 12, 2011, accessed July 24, 2012, www.cdc.gov/heartdisease/aspirin.htm.
- Giorgia De Berardis et al., "Association of Aspirin Use with Major Bleeding in Patients with and Without Diabetes," *Journal of the American Medical Association* 307 (June 6, 2012): 2286–94.

40. Are Name-Brand Drugs Better than Generic?

- "What Are Generic Drugs?," Food and Drug Administration, last modified May 12, 2009, accessed November 9, 2012, www.fda.gov/Drugs/ResourcesForYou/Consumers/BuyingUsing MedicineSafely/UnderstandingGenericDrugs/ucm144456.htm.

41. Can I Use a Drug After the Expiration Date?

- "Audit of the Shelf Life Extension Program (SLEP) at the Centers for Disease Control and Prevention," Office of Inspector General, U.S. Department of Health and Human Services, August 2011, www.oig.hhs.gov/oas/reports/region4/41101001.pdf.
- "Pharmaceutical Expiration Dates," Reports of Council on Scientific Affairs, American Medical Association, June 2001, 401–406, www.ama-assn.org/meetings/public/annual01/csa _reports.pdf#search%C2%BC%E2%80%98Pharmaceutical%20Expiration%20Dates.

42. Are Over-the-Counter Pain Relievers Interchangeable?

- American Academy of Family Physicians and American Pharmacists Association, "Appropriate Use of Common OTC Analgesics and Cough and Cold Medications," October 2008, www.aafp.org/online/etc/medialib/aafp_org/documents/news_pubs/mono/otc.Par.0001.File .tmp/OTCmonograph.pdf.
- "Aspirin: Questions and Answers," Information for Consumers, U.S. Food and Drug Administration, last modified August 8, 2011, accessed November 9, 2012, www.fda.gov /Drugs/ResourcesForYou/Consumers/QuestionsAnswers/ucm071879.htm.
- "The Benefits and Risks of Pain Relievers: Q&A with Sharon Hertz, M.D.," Consumer Health Information, U.S. Food and Drug Administration, April 26, 2007, www.fda.gov /downloads/ForConsumers/ConsumerUpdates/ucm107859.pdf.
- "Acetaminophen and Liver Injury: Q&A for Consumers," Consumer Updates, U.S. Food and Drug Administration, last modified August 9, 2012, accessed November 9, 2012, www .fda.gov/ForConsumers/ConsumerUpdates/ucm168830.htm.
- "Pain relief guide: What to Take When with So Many Choices, Here's How to Figure It Out," ConsumerReports.org, last modified April 2011, accessed November 9, 2012, www .consumerreports.org/cro/2012/04/pain-relief-guide-what-to-take-when/index.htm.

43. Are Herbal Supplements as Effective as Other Medications?

- National Center for Complementary and Alternative Medicine, National Institutes of Health, nccam.nih.gov/.
- "Tips for the Savvy Supplement User: Making Informed Decisions and Evaluating Information," Consumer Information, U.S. Food and Drug Administration, last modified October 9, 2012, accessed November 9, 2012, www.fda.gov/Food/DietarySupplements/ConsumerInformation/ucm110567.htm.
- "Dietary Supplements—Q&A," Consumer Information, U.S. Food and Drug Administration, last modified September 4, 2012, accessed November 9, 2012, www.fda.gov/Food/DietarySupplements/ConsumerInformation/ucm191930.htm.
- "Dietary Supplements: What You Need to Know," Food Facts, U.S. Food and Drug Administration, last modified January 26, 2012, accessed November 9, 2012, www.fda.gov/Food/ResourcesForYou/Consumers/ucm109760.htm.
- Jaime Gahche et al., "Dietary Supplement Use Among U.S. Adults Has Increased Since NHANES III (1988–1994)," NCHS Data Brief, no 61, National Center for Health Statistics, 2011, www.cdc.gov/nchs/data/databriefs/db61.pdf.
- Michael Spector, *Denialism: How Irrational Thinking Hinders Scientific Progress, Harms the Planet, and Threatens Our Lives* (New York: Penguin Press, 2009).
- "Does Airborne Really Stave Off Colds?," *Good Morning America,* ABC News, February 27, 2006, abcnews.go.com/GMA/OnCall/story?id=1664514&page=1#.UEI0YqThdlY.
- Ronald B. Turner et al., "An Evaluation of *Echinacea angustifolia* in Experimental Rhinovirus Infections," *New England Journal of Medicine* 353 (July 28, 2005): 341–48.
- Klaus Linde et al., "Echinacea for Preventing and Treating the Common Cold," *Cochrane Database of Systematic Reviews* 2006, Issue 1, Art. No. CD000530.
- Federal Trade Commission. "Makers of Airborne Settle FTC Charges of Deceptive Advertising; Agreement Brings Total Settlement Funds to $30 Million" August 14, 2008, www.ftc.gov/opa/2008/08/airborne.shtm

44. What Are the Most Dangerous Drugs?

- "Prescription Drugs," National Institute on Drug Abuse, National Institutes of Health, accessed November 11, 2012, www.drugabuse.gov/drugs-abuse/prescription-drugs.
- "Unintentional Poisoning," Centers for Disease Control and Prevention, last modified July 11, 2012, accessed November 11, 2012, www.cdc.gov/homeandrecreationalsafety/pdf/poison-issue-brief.pdf.
- "Prevent Unintentional Poisoning," CDC Features, Centers for Disease Control and Prevention, last modified March 19, 2012, accessed November 11, 2012, www.cdc.gov/Features/PoisonPrevention/.
- Margaret Warner et al., "Drug Poisoning Deaths in the United States, 1980–2008," NCHS Data Brief, no 81, National Center for Health Statistics, December 2011, www.cdc.gov/nchs/data/databriefs/db81.htm.
- "McNeil Consumer Healthcare Announces Plans for New Dosing Instructions for Tylenol Products," Johnson & Johnson, July 28, 2011, accessed November 11, 2012, www.jnj.com/connect/news/all/mcneil-consumer-healthcare-announces-plans-for-new-dosing-instructions-for-tylenol-products.

- Press release, "Too Much of a Good Thing: Expert Warns of Overuse of Over-the-Counter Pain Medication," University of Michigan Health System, March 6, 2006, accessed November 11, 2012, www.med.umich.edu/opm/newspage/2006/hmotc.htm.
- "Acetaminophen Overdose," MedlinePlus, U.S. National Library of Medicine and National Institutes of Health, accessed November 11, 2012, www.nlm.nih.gov/medlineplus/ency/article/002598.htm.

45. Should I Take a Statin to Prevent High Cholesterol?
- "Cholesterol: What You Can Do," Centers for Disease Control and Prevention, last modified March 14, 2012, accessed November 11, 2012, www.cdc.gov/cholesterol/what_you_can_do.htm.
- "Risk Assessment Tool for Estimating 10-Year Risk of Having a Heart Attack," National Cholesterol Education Program, Third Report of the Expert Panel on Detection, Evaluation, and Treatment of High Blood Cholesterol in Adults (Adult Treatment Panel III), accessed November 11, 2012, hp2010.nhlbihin.net/atpIII/calculator.asp.
- "ATP III AT-A-Glance: Quick Desk Reference," National Cholesterol Education Program, Third Report of the Expert Panel on Detection, Evaluation, and Treatment of High Blood Cholesterol in Adults (Adult Treatment Panel III), NIH Publication No. 01-3305, May 2001, accessed November 11, 2012, www.nhlbi.nih.gov/guidelines/cholesterol/atglance.htm.

46. Should I Use Hormone Therapy for My Menopause Symptoms?
- Writing Group for the Women's Health Initiative Investigators, "Risks and Benefits of Estrogen Plus Progestin in Healthy Postmenopausal Women: Principal Results from the Women's Health Initiative Randomized Controlled Trial," *Journal of the American Medical Association* 288 (July 17, 2002): 321–33.
- "Facts About Menopausal Hormone Therapy," National Institutes of Health, NIH Publication No. 05-5200, last modified June 2005, accessed November 11, 2012, www.nhlbi.nih.gov/health/women/pht_facts.pdf.
- "Menopausal Hormone Therapy," Womenshealth.gov, U.S. Department of Health and Human Services Office on Women's Health, last modified September 29, 2010, accessed November 11, 2012, www.womenshealth.gov/menopause/symptom-relief-treatment/menopausal-hormone-therapy.cfm.
- U.S. Preventive Services Task Force, "Hormone Therapy for the Prevention of Chronic Conditions in Postmenopausal Women: Recommendation Statement," AHRQ Publication No. 05-0576, May 2005, accessed November 11, 2012, www.uspreventiveservicestaskforce.org/uspstf05/ht/htpostmenrs.htm.

47. Should I Take Calcium for Stronger Bones?
- "Calculation Tool," FRAX, WHO [World Health Organization] Fracture Risk Assessment Tool, accessed November 11, 2012, www.shef.ac.uk/FRAX/tool.jsp?country=9.
- U.S. Preventive Services Task Force, "Vitamin D and Calcium Supplementation to Prevent Cancer and Osteoporotic Fractures in Adults: Draft Recommendation Statement," AHRQ Publication No. 12-05163-EF-2, June 12, 2012, accessed November 11, 2012, www.uspreventiveservicestaskforce.org/uspstf12/vitamind/draftrecvitd.htm.
- U.S. Preventive Services Task Force, "Screening for Osteoporosis: Recommendation

Statement," AHRQ Publication No. 10-05145-EF-2, January 2011, accessed November 11, 2012, www.uspreventiveservicestaskforce.org/uspstf10/osteoporosis/osteors.htm.

- Jaime Gahche et al., "Dietary Supplement Use Among U.S. Adults Has Increased Since NHANES III (1988–1994)," NCHS Data Brief, No. 61, National Center for Health Statistics, 2011, www.cdc.gov/nchs/data/databriefs/db61.pdf.
- "Dietary Reference Intakes for Calcium and Vitamin D," Institute of Medicine, last modified December 1, 2012, accessed November 11, 2012, www.iom.edu/Reports/2010/Dietary -Reference-Intakes-for-Calcium-and-Vitamin-D/DRI-Values.aspx.
- "Calcium and Vitamin D: What You Need to Know," National Osteoporosis Foundation, accessed November 11, 2012, www.nof.org/aboutosteoporosis/prevention/calcium.

48. Where Should I Store Medications?

- "Poisoning in the United States: Fact Sheet," Centers for Disease Control and Prevention, last modified June 29, 2012, accessed November 9, 2012, www.cdc.gov/homeandrecreationalsafety /poisoning/poisoning-factsheet.htm.
- "Preventing Children from Getting into 'Child-Resistant' Medicine Bottles," *World News with Diane Sawyer*, ABC News, December 24, 2009, abcnews.go.com/WN/abcs-dr-richard besser-kids-child-resistant-medicine/story?id=9420083.
- "Toddler Poisoned by Prescriptions," *Good Morning America*, ABC News, December 20, 2010, abcnews.go.com/Health/Wellness/children-overdose-parents-medications /story?id=12423751.

Chapter 5:   An Ounce of Prevention, A Pound of Cure: Your Questions for Understanding, Preventing, and Responding to Illness and Injury

49. Can I Catch the Same Infection Twice?

- "How Vaccines Prevent Disease," Centers for Disease Control and Prevention, last modified April 25, 2012, accessed November 11, 2012, www.cdc.gov/vaccines/vac-gen /howvpd.htm.
- "Understanding the Immune System: How It Works," National Institutes of Health, NIH Publication No. 07-5423, September 2007, accessed November 11, 2012, www.niaid.nih.gov /topics/immuneSystem/Documents/theimmunesystem.pdf.

50. Is Rest the Best Thing for Back Pain?

- "Low Back Pain Fact Sheet," National Institutes of Health, last modified September 19, 2012, accessed November 11, 2012, www.ninds.nih.gov/disorders/backpain/detail_backpain.htm.
- Antti Malmivaara et al., "The Treatment of Acute Low Back Pain—Bed Rest, Exercises, or Ordinary Activity?," *New England Journal of Medicine* 332 (February 9, 1995): 351–55.

51. If No One in My Family Has Had Breast Cancer, Can I Still Get It?

- "Breast Cancer Facts & Figures 2011–2012," American Cancer Society, 2011, www.cancer.org /acs/groups/content/@epidemiologysurveilance/documents/document/acspc-030975.pdf.
- "Estimated New Cancer Cases and Deaths for 2012: All Races, By Sex; SEER Cancer

Statistics Review 1975–2009," "Cancer Facts & Figures–2012," American Cancer Society, 2012, seer.cancer.gov/csr/1975_2009_pops09/results_single/sect_01_table.01.pdf.

- "Women's Health USA 2011—Cancer," U.S. Department of Health and Human Services, Health Resources and Services Administration, 2011, accessed November 11, 2012, mchb .hrsa.gov/whusa11/hstat/hshi/pages/214c.html.
- Lori Mosca et al., "National Study of Women's Awareness, Preventive Action, and Barriers to Cardiovascular Health," *Circulation* 113 (January 31, 2006): 525–534.
- "Go Red for Women: About the Movement," American Heart Association, accessed November 11, 2012, www.goredforwomen.org/about_the_movement.aspx.
- U.S. Preventive Services Task Force, "Screening for Breast Cancer: Recommendation Statement," AHRQ Publication No. 10-05142-EF-2, November 2009, accessed November 12, 2012, www.uspreventiveservicestaskforce.org/uspstf09/breastcancer/brcanrs.htm.
- "U.S. Breast Cancer Statistics," Breastcancer.org, last modified October 30, 2012, accessed November 12, 2012, www.breastcancer.org/symptoms/understand_bc/statistics.jsp.
- "Genetics," BreastCancer.org, last modified September 17, 2012, accessed November 12, 2012, www.breastcancer.org/risk/factors/genetics.jsp.
- Wendy Y. Chen et al., "Moderate Alcohol Consumption During Adult Life, Drinking Patterns, and Breast Cancer Risk," *Journal of the American Medical Association* 306 (November 2, 2011): 1884–90.
- Fei Xue et al., "Cigarette Smoking and the Incidence of Breast Cancer," *Archives of Internal Medicine* 171 (January 2011): 125–33.
- D. M. Parkin, "Cancers Attributable to Inadequate Physical Exercise in the UK in 2010," *British Journal of Cancer* 105 (December 2011): S38–S41; "Factsheet: Menopausal Hormone Therapy and Cancer," National Cancer Institute, reviewed December 5, 2011, accessed November 12, 2012, www.cancer.gov/cancertopics/factsheet/Risk/menopausal-hormones.

52. Are Heart Attack Symptoms the Same in Men and Women?

- "1 Am Women Heart: The National Coalition for Women with Heart Disease," accessed November 12, 2012, www.womenheart.org/.
- "Subtle and Dangerous: Symptoms of Heart Disease in Women," National Institute of Nursing Research, National Institutes of Health, 2006, NIH Publication No. 06-6079, www .ninr.nih.gov/NR/rdonlyres/054108E8-E4A3-4A09-AA0C-E56D2A09F411/0/NIN-RHEART1216062508.pdf.
- "Women and Heart Disease Fact Sheet," Centers for Disease Control and Prevention, last modified October 18, 2012, accessed November 12, 2012, www.cdc.gov/dhdsp/data_statistics /fact_sheets/fs_women_heart.htm.

53. Can I Call In Sick with a Cold?

- "Common Cold," National Institutes of Health, last modified August 17, 2011, accessed November 12, 2012, www.niaid.nih.gov/topics/commoncold/Pages/default.aspx.
- Press release, "National Survey Finds Six in Ten Americans Believe Serious Outbreak of Influenza A (H1N1) Likely in Fall/Winter," Harvard School of Public Health, July 15, 2009, accessed November 12, 2012, www.hsph.harvard.edu/news/press-releases/2009-releases /national-survey-americans-influenza-a-h1n1-outbreak-fall-winter.html.

54. Can I Die of a Broken Heart?

- Ilan S. Wittstein et al., "Neurohumoral Features of Myocardial Stunning Due to Sudden Emotional Stress," *New England Journal of Medicine* 352 (February 10, 2005): 539–48.

55. Do Cell Phones Cause Brain Cancer?

- "Cellular Phones," American Cancer Society, last modified February 23, 2012, accessed November 12, 2012, www.cancer.org/Cancer/CancerCauses/OtherCarcinogens/AtHome/cellular-phones.
- "Factsheet: Cell Phones and Cancer Risk," National Cancer Institute, reviewed June 18, 2012, accessed November 12, 2012, www.cancer.gov/cancertopics/factsheet/Risk/cellphones.
- Nora D. Volkow et al., "Effects of Cell Phone Radiofrequency Signal Exposure on Brain Glucose Metabolism," *Journal of the American Medical Association* 305 (February 23, 2011): 808–13.
- Interphone Study Group, "Brain Tumour Risk in Relation to Mobile Telephone Use: Results of the INTERPHONE International Case–Control Study," *International Journal of Epidemiology* 39 (May 17, 2010): 675–94.
- Governors Highway Safety Association, "Distracted Driving: What Research Shows and What States Can Do," 2011, accessed November 12, 2011, www.ghsa.org/html/publications/pdf/sfdist11.pdf.
- David L. Strayer, Frank A. Drews, and Dennis J. Crouch, "A Comparison of the Cell Phone Driver and the Drunk Driver," *Human Factors: The Journal of the Human Factors and Ergonomics Society* 48 (Summer 2006): 381–391.
- Experian Simmons, "The 2011 Mobile Consumer Report," www.experian.com/assets/simmons-research/white-papers/experian-simmons-2011-mobile-consumer-report.pdf.

56. What Should I Do If I Think I'm Having a Stroke?

- "Warning Signs of Stroke," National Stroke Association, accessed November 12, 2012, www.stroke.org/site/PageServer?pagename=SYMP.
- "Stroke Facts," Centers for Disease Control and Prevention, last modified October 17, 2012, accessed November 12, 2012, www.cdc.gov/stroke/facts.htm.
- National Institute of Neurological Disorders and Stroke rt-PA Stroke Study Group, "Tissue Plasminogen Activator for Acute Ischemic Stroke," *New England Journal of Medicine* 333 (December 14, 1995): 1581–88.

57. Should I Be Worried if I'm Shaped like an Apple?

- Sarah Camhi, JoAnn Kuo, and Deborah R. Young, "Identifying Adolescent Metabolic Syndrome Using Body Mass Index and Waist Circumference," *Preventing Chronic Disease* 5 (October 2008), www.cdc.gov/pcd/issues/2008/oct/07_0170.htm.

Chapter 6:   Take Control of Your Health: Your Questions on
How to Avoid Getting Overtested, Overtreated, and Harmed by Health Care

59. How Do I Stay Safe in the Hospital?

- Office of the Inspector General, U.S. Department of Health and Human Services, "Adverse Events in Hospitals: National Incidence among Medicare Beneficiaries," Report OEI-06-09-00090, November 2010, https://oig.hhs.gov/oei/reports/oei-06-09-00090.pdf.
- "20 Tips to Help Prevent Medical Errors—Patient Fact Sheet," Agency for Healthcare Research and Quality, AHRQ Publication No. 11-0089, last reviewed September 2011, accessed November 12, 2012, www.ahrq.gov/consumer/20tips.htm.
- "Patient Safety: Ten Things You Can Do to Be a Safe Patient," Centers for Disease Control and Prevention, last modified February 3, 2011, accessed November 12, 2012, www.cdc.gov/HAI/patientSafety/patient-safety.html.
- "Hospital Ratings," ConsumerReports.org, accessed November 12, 2012, www.consumer reports.org/health/doctors-hospitals/hospital-ratings/ratings/search-results.htm (subscription required).
- "Hospital Compare," Medicare.gov, U.S. Department of Health and Human Services, last modified October 11, 2012, accessed November 12, 2012, www.hospitalcompare.hhs.gov.

60. Does Where My Doctor Went to Medical School Matter?

- Rachel O. Reid et al., "Associations Between Physician Characteristics and Quality of Care," *Archives of Internal Medicine* 170 (September 2010): 1442–49.
- "Choosing a Primary Care Provider," MedlinePlus, U.S. National Library of Medicine and National Institutes of Health, last modified January 23, 2012, accessed November 12, 2012, www.nlm.nih.gov/medlineplus/ency/article/001939.htm.
- "Medical School Admissions Statistics & Trends," Office of Pre Professional Programs and Advising, Johns Hopkins University, accessed November 12, 2012, web.jhu.edu/prepro/health/admissions_stats.html.
- "Choosing a Doctor," Agency for Healthcare Research and Quality (archive), accessed November 12, 2012, archive.ahrq.gov/consumer/qnt/qntdr.htm.
- Association of American Medical Colleges, "Medical School Graduation and Attrition Rates," *Analysis in Brief* 7 (April 2007), accessed November 12, 2012, www.aamc.org/download/102346/data/aibvol7no2.pdf.
- Katy Hopkins, "10 Medical Schools with Lowest Acceptance Rates," *U.S. News & World Report*, April 5, 2011, accessed November 12, 2012, www.usnews.com/education/best-graduate-schools/articles/2011/04/05/10-medical-schools-with-lowest-acceptance-rates.

61. Should I Get an Annual Physical?

- "Guide to Clinical Preventive Services, 2010-2011—Preventive Services Recommended by the USPSTF," Agency for Healthcare Research and Quality, accessed November 12, 2012, www.ahrq.gov/clinic/pocketgd1011/gcp10s1.htm.
- "Men: Stay Healthy at Any Age," AHRQ Publication No. 10-IP004-A, September 2010, Agency for Healthcare Research and Quality, accessed November 12, 2012, www.ahrq.gov/ppip/healthymen.htm.

- "Women: Stay Healthy at Any Age," AHRQ Publication No. 10-IP002-A, September 2010, Agency for Healthcare Research and Quality, accessed November 12, 2012, www.ahrq.gov /ppip/healthywom.htm.

62. Should I Ask for a Second Opinion?

- "Getting a Second Opinion Before Surgery," Centers for Medicare & Medicaid Services, U.S. Department of Health and Human Services, CMS Product No. 02173, last updated June 2010, accessed November 13, 2012, www.medicare.gov/publications/pubs/pdf/02173.pdf.
- "How to Get a Second Opinion," National Women's Health Information Center, U.S. Department of Health and Human Services, last updated September 10, 2008, accessed November 13, 2012, womenshealth.gov/publications/our-publications/second-opinion-how-to.pdf.
- Rick Blizzard, "First Opinion Good Enough for Most Patients," Gallup, June 7, 2005, accessed November 13, 2012, www.gallup.com/poll/16654/first-opinion-good-enough-most -patients.aspx.

63. If My Doctors Order a Lot of Tests, Does That Mean They're More Thorough?

- "Five Things Physicians and Patients Should Question," Choosing Wisely: An Initiative of the ABIM Foundation, accessed November 13, 2012, choosingwisely.org/?page_id=13.
- Martin M. Oken et al., for the PLCO Project Team, "Screening by Chest Radiograph and Lung Cancer Mortality: The Prostate, Lung, Colorectal, and Ovarian (PLCO) Randomized Trial," *Journal of the American Medical Association* 306 (November 2, 2011): 1865–73.

64. Is the Internet a Good Place to Get Medical Information?

- Susannah Fox, "The Social Life of Health Information," Pew Research Center, Internet & American Life Project, May 12, 2011, accessed November 13, 2012, pewresearch.org /pubs/1989/health-care-online-social-network-users.

65. Are Genetic Tests Effective?

- U.S. Government Accountability Office, "Misleading Test Results Are Further Complicated by Deceptive Marketing and Other Questionable Practices," GAO-10-847T, July 22, 2010, www.gao.gov/products/GAO-10-847T.
- "Adult Family History Form," American Medical Association, accessed November 13, 2012, www.ama-assn.org/resources/doc/genetics/adult_history.pdf.
- "My Family Health Portrait: A Tool from the Surgeon General," U.S. Department of Health and Human Services, accessed November 13, 2012, familyhistory.hhs.gov/fhh-web/home. action.

66. Does a PSA Test Accurately Detect Prostate Cancer?

- Virginia A. Moyer, on behalf of the U.S. Preventive Services Task Force, "Screening for Prostate Cancer: U.S. Preventive Services Task Force Recommendation Statement," *Annals of Internal Medicine* 157 (July 17, 2012): 120–34.
- "Prostate Cancer Screening." National Cancer Institute, last modified October 5, 2012, accessed November 13, 2012, www.cancer.gov/cancertopics/pdq/screening/prostate/Health- Professional/page2.

- American Urological Association, "Prostate-Specific Antigen Best Practice Statement: 2009 Update," 2009, accessed November 13, 2012, www.auanet.org/content/media/psa09.pdf.
- Andrew M. D. Wolf et al., "American Cancer Society Guideline for the Early Detection of Prostate Cancer: Update 2010," *Cancer: A Cancer Journal for Clinicians* 60 (March/April 2010): 70–98.
- Richard J. Albin, "The Great Prostate Mistake," *New York Times*, March 9, 2010, www .nytimes.com/2010/03/10/opinion/10Ablin.html?_r=1.
- Richard M. Martin, "Commentary: Prostate Cancer Is Omnipresent, but Should We Screen for It?," *International Journal of Epidemiology* 36 (April 2007): 278–81.

67. Should I Get Dental X-Rays Every Year?

- "Reducing Radiation from Medical X-Rays," U.S. Food and Drug Administration, last modified August 9, 2012, accessed November 13, 2012, www.fda.gov/ForConsumers /ConsumerUpdates/ucm095505.htm.
- American Dental Association Council on Scientific Affairs, "The Use of Dental Radiographs: Update and Recommendations," *Journal of the American Dental Association* 137 (September 2006): 1304–12.

68. Are Hospitals More Dangerous in July?

- John Q. Young et al., "'July Effect': Impact of the Academic Year-End Changeover on Patient Outcomes: A Systematic Review," *Annals of Internal Medicine* 155 (September 6, 2011): 309–15.
- Office of the Inspector General, U.S. Department of Health and Human Services, "Hospital Incident Reporting Systems Do Not Capture Most Patient Harm," Report (OEI-06-09-00091), January 5, 2012, oig.hhs.gov/oei/reports/oei-06-09-00091.asp.
- "20 Tips to Help Prevent Medical Errors—Patient Fact Sheet," Agency for Healthcare Research and Quality, AHRQ Publication No. 11-0089, last modified September 2011, accessed November 13, 2012, www.ahrq.gov/consumer/20tips.htm.

INDEX